A Woman's Guide to a Healthy Heart

Carol Simontacchi, C.C.N., M.S.,
and Frances E. FitzGerald

Contemporary Books

Chicago   New York   San Francisco   Lisbon   London   Madrid   Mexico City
Milan   New Delhi   San Juan   Seoul   Singapore   Sydney   Toronto

1 2 3 4 5 6 7 8 9 0   DOC/DOC   2 1 0 9 8 7 6 5 4 3

ISBN 0-658-02158-3

Interior design by Robert S. Tinnon

McGraw-Hill books are available at special quantity discounts to use as premiums and
sales promotions, or for use in corporate training programs. For more information, please
write to the Director of Special Sales, Professional Publishing, McGraw-Hill, Two Penn
Plaza, New York, NY 10121-2298. Or contact your local bookstore.

This book is printed on acid-free paper.

Contents

Introduction

Press your ear against the breast of a woman and hear her heartbeat: Rhythmic, strong, warm.

Describe her heart. It is about the size of her closed hand. It weighs about 300 grams (10 ounces) and is cone shaped—not shaped like a valentine! It lies in the center of her chest, nestled between the left and right lungs. Blood rushing through the vessels stain the tissues crimson red. It pulses in a double rhythm: once as the blood is pushed out of the heart to circulate throughout the body, and once as the blood is pushed back into the heart.

The heart is the center of the cardiovascular system, a vast network of arteries, veins, and capillaries that feed every cell in the body. It never rests, except for a brief millisecond between the pulses. It pumps more than thirty times its own weight in blood each minute, more than 1,800 gallons of blood a day, and over 1.3 million gallons a year.

The heart works this hard when the woman is sitting or lying down. When she is active (and what woman isn't?), it works even harder.

But the physical details pale before the spiritual description of her heart. We speak of this physical organ in clichés: "You're all heart," "Have a heart," "Don't break my heart," "I love you with all of my heart," "My heart wasn't in it."

We understand these trite phrases. We know we're not speaking of the 300-gram organ that pumps life throughout the body. We're speaking of something deeper—we're speaking of the heart as a nontangible receptacle of our emotions, as the center of our emotional being. When we speak of the heart, we think of the feelings we share with other people. Our hearts are our emotional core.

Positive feelings such as love, trust, and gratitude can nourish the heart. In this book, we'll see that this is true physically as well as metaphorically.

Conversely, negative emotions such as loneliness, sadness, and resentment can break both the physical and the emotional heart.

Women are particularly vulnerable to the effects of positive and negative emotions, especially on the health of their cardiovascular systems. So when we talk of nourishing the female heart, we'll discuss how to sustain the emotional heart as well as the physical one. We'll talk about how our postmodern culture is as emotionally deprived as it is nutritionally deprived—and how to restore that emotional and nutritional richness.

Science is now catching up to what poets have known for centuries: emotions can break—and heal—hearts. In one study, patients with coronary artery disease filled out questionnaires about their emotional lives. They also underwent an angiogram. Two years later, 150 of the patients underwent a second angiogram. In those who scored high on anger and low on social support, the progression of the disease was significantly greater than the other patients in the study, independent of medication or other risk factors.[1]

Depression is another risk factor for heart disease. In a study of elderly women, those with the highest scores for depression had a 40 percent increased risk of heart disease, and 60 percent faced an increased risk of death.[2]

Do depression and other painful emotions lead to illness, or does illness lead to painful emotions? Women with hypertension (high blood pressure) are far more likely to suffer from depression, and depression is a major risk factor for heart disease. The yet-unanswered question is, Which comes first, the depression or the high blood pressure?[3]

Stress is also hard on the heart. The author of one study noted, "It is known that mental stress can impair the endothelium, the protective barrier lining the blood vessels."[4]

Female participants in another study reported whether they felt they were high or low on the social ladder. The women who perceived themselves as being on the low end of the social ladder experienced more stress. These women secreted more of a stress hormone called cortisol. Cortisol appears to contribute to the buildup of abdominal fat—a risk factor for heart disease.[5] In addition, cortisol increases blood pressure, deregulates blood sugar, and causes psychological changes such as depression—all risk factors for heart disease. Furthermore, excessive secretion of cortisol affects every other organ of the endocrine system, including the thyroid gland, as well as the steroid hormones such as estrogen, progesterone, and testosterone.

We know certain emotions—anger, loneliness, and stress—cause plenty of wear and tear on the heart. What about positive emotions, such as mirth?

Humor may reduce your risk of heart disease. Researchers pulled together three hundred individuals to learn how they deal with stressful situations, and found that "heart-healthy people are more likely than those with heart disease to laugh frequently and heartily." In one study, 150 people who had suffered heart attacks or who had undergone heart bypass surgery were compared with healthy individuals with no history of heart disease. Researchers found that healthy people were more likely to laugh often and use humor to get out of uncomfortable situations. On the other hand, those with heart disease were not able to laugh their way out of embarrassing moments.

Those with the highest "humor scores" had a 48 percent lower risk of heart disease, independent of their age or gender. Dr. Miller, one of the authors of the study, noted, "Exactly how laughter may protect the heart isn't entirely understood . . . but some evidence suggests that the effects of a chortle, snicker, or guffaw include reduction in stress hormones such as cortisol, and reduction in blood pressure. That in turn may reduce heart disease risk."[6] By the way, the researchers found that laughing with a friend was even more protective than laughing alone! (In Chapter 4, we'll discuss in greater detail the impact of emotions on a woman's heart.)

We Aren't Eating Well, Either

The health of our hearts is influenced by nutrition as well as emotions. As a culture, we are nutritionally bankrupt, or nearly so. That is an amazing fact to ponder, considering that we are swimming in a sea of information and interest in health and nutrition that is at an all-time high. Supermarket shelves are awash in so-called healthy products.

Study after study, however, shows that the average American is deficient in numerous nutrients, all of which are critically important to the heart. Some "experts" assure us that we are living longer and therefore are healthier. But other pundits remark that it is simply taking us longer to die, and increasing numbers of Americans are struggling with chronic debilitating diseases that could be avoided if we simply ate (and lived) better. Heart disease is one of those chronic debilitating illnesses that is directly affected by what we eat.

The Number-One Cause of Death

Heart disease has primarily been considered a male problem and, as a result, many women underestimate their risk of dying of heart attack and/or stroke (another form of cardiovascular illness). In fact, heart disease is the leading killer of women, with an estimated 500,000 deaths each year.

Approximately 25 percent of women have blood cholesterol levels high enough to pose a serious risk for heart disease. Blood cholesterol among women tends to rise sharply beginning at the age of forty until the age of sixty. Fifty percent of women over the age of fifty-five are at risk of heart disease because of high blood pressure alone.[7]

While increasing age is a risk factor for cardiovascular disease, no woman should feel that she is immune. One in ten American women aged forty-five to sixty-four has some form of heart disease. This figure increases to one in five women after age sixty-five. Stroke occurs in another 1.6 million American women each year.

We've Been Left Out

The statistics on women and heart disease are sobering. Until recently, however, this area of scientific study has been largely ignored. While billions of dollars have been spent trying to understand the cause and cure of heart disease in men, little money has been expended to try to answer the same question for women. Researchers solicited thousands of men for their projects, and ignored the other half of society. They then extrapolated their findings to the female population, even though women's physiology is much different from men's.

Why were women excluded from pharmaceutical trials that might have yielded valuable information on a life-threatening illness? Researchers were concerned about the possibility of birth defects in younger women. Women who were postmenopausal, who had undergone a hysterectomy, or who were using estrogen replacement therapy were also excluded, however. Researchers feared that fluctuations in estrogen and progesterone levels would impair the effectiveness of the drugs under study.

Other cardiovascular studies initially included men but omitted research findings from the data reports. Yet findings from these studies were broadly applied to women, despite their very different hormonal influences.

The Nurses' Health Study, started in 1976, included 121,700 female nurses; it was the first study of this magnitude to focus on heart disease and other health issues specifically in women. Since the Nurses' Health Study began, women's health has become the focus of increased research.

The NIH (National Institutes of Health) Revitalization Act of 1993 provided updated guidelines regarding this issue. The NIH is now required to include women and minorities in clinical studies.[8]

Heart Disease in Women and in Men

Women do not fare as well as men in the event of a cardiovascular event. For example, women who undergo surgery for heart disease generally have a poorer prognosis than do men. Other studies have shown that women have a worse outcome than men following a first myocardial infarction (heart attack), even after controlling for potentially confounding factors such as smoking, diabetes, high blood pressure, previous angina (heart pain), time to admission to a cardiovascular hospital unit, and treatment choice.

Part of the reason for the poorer prognosis may be that women simply don't get to the hospital as quickly as men once they suspect they are in physical trouble. It may take up to one hour longer for women to check themselves into an emergency room after the first symptoms of a heart attack. Why is that? Women simply may not put "heart attack" on their list of possibilities once they begin to experience the ominous symptoms. Another explanation may be that women are accustomed to caring for others before they take care of themselves.

In addition, the delay between the emergency room visit and admission to the coronary care unit is also significantly longer in women (9.3 versus 7 hours). This may be explained by the fact that even hospital staff members don't think "heart attack" when they see the less obvious signs of a cardiovascular event in a woman. That small distinction of more than one hour may mean the difference between life and death.

The twenty-eight day mortality rate and the six-month readmission and mortality rates have been significantly higher in women than in men. This difference is due to the more severe acute myocardial infarction (AMI) rather than a woman's history of cardiovascular risk factors, comorbidity (another disease that coexists with coronary artery disease), or thrombolytic treatment (to break up blood clots). Women experience other differences in cardiovascular events as well:

- Women usually develop coronary artery disease (CAD) about ten years later than men.
- High triglyceride levels ("good" cholesterol) and low HDL levels confer a greater CAD risk in women than men.
- Diabetes is a greater risk factor for women than for men.
- Smoking increases CAD risk and negates the protective effects of estrogen in women.

No matter how you tell the tale, heart disease is certainly a woman's issue, and nearly always results in a worse conclusion for women than for men. (See Chapter 1 for more information about the medical disparity between women and men.)

Educational Factors

Can a college education reduce your risk of heart disease? A study in Sweden suggests that it does. The study included 292 women with coronary heart disease (CHD) with 292 age-matched controls. After adjusting for psychosocial stress, unhealthy lifestyle patterns, high blood pressure, and lipid profile (fats in the blood), researchers found a greater risk of CHD in women with less education. The authors of the study concluded, "The increased risk of CHD in women with low education appears to be linked to psychosocial stress and lifestyle factors. . . . These factors may be considered in strategies geared toward reducing socioeconomic inequalities in cardiovascular health."[9]

Specifically, the risk of CHD is about twice as high in women with less than or equal to a high school education, compared with women who have a college degree. Women with less education also have increased rates of smoking, obesity, high blood pressure, and high cholesterol levels, as well as poor coping skills, social isolation, and job stress. Women with more education are likely to be able to take control of their lives, thus reducing stress levels, and have a greater chance of enjoying the company of other women in similar situations—another positive in terms of stress reduction.

We'll explore lifestyle issues later in this book. Keep in mind, however, that women with college degrees are more likely to enjoy higher-paying jobs and have more time to take care of themselves physically, spiritually, socially, and emotionally.

Other Risk Factors

While emotions play a large role in the health of the cardiovascular system, they aren't the only factor. Some intensely hostile individuals sail through life with nary a care about heart disease, and die of a ripe old age from other causes. (Some people would say they *cause* heart disease, they don't *get* it!) Some well-adjusted, good-natured women crumple from heart disease at an early age, leaving their bewildered families bereft of their cheery dispositions.

We can increase our risk of heart disease by poor lifestyle choices. These are purely physical in nature. For example, nearly one-fifth of deaths from cardiovascular diseases are attributed to smoking, either one's own or someone else's. About 37,000 to 40,000 nonsmokers die each year from cardiovascular diseases, simply because they live or work with a smoker. They increase their risk of heart disease by breathing in secondhand smoke.

Approximately 96 million American women and men have blood cholesterol levels of 200 mg/dL and higher. About 37.8 million American adults have levels of 240 or above. An estimated 24 percent of Americans aged eighteen or older report no leisure-time physical activity. Inactivity is a risk factor in heart disease, comparable to high cholesterol, high blood pressure, and smoking.

Nutritional deficiencies have been implicated in heart disease. Some of the most well-known cardiovascular-supporting nutrients are coenzyme Q10, calcium, magnesium, several of the B complex vitamins, vitamin C, copper, potassium, and selenium. We'll find out in Chapter 5 that significant numbers of Americans (particularly dieting American women) are deficient in most of these nutrients.

How Our Modern Lives Contribute to Heart Disease

The shelves of American supermarkets are bulging with an abundance of food, and yet we suffer from chronic malnutrition. How is this possible?

The standard American diet (SAD) is high in fat and sodium and low in the nutrients listed above. With our growing awareness of the need for healthy foods, why are we eating so poorly? Quite bluntly, we have lost our meaningful relationships with our pots and pans. We have no time to prepare home-cooked meals, and we depend on restaurants and fast-food joints to feed us. In fact, the total receipts for the restaurant sector in the second quarter of 2001 added up to $13.9 billion. While restaurant meals may be large, they often don't feed us well. Want a nearly out-of-body eating experience? Just drop by one of the thousands of restaurants lining the highways and sample their fare; you'll quickly discover just how terrible our American food really is. It doesn't taste good, and it is bad for the heart.

The second major culprit is the diet industry. Promoters of unhealthy fad diets reap a fortune from the desperation of people who believe they can't lose weight any other way. Which diet is unhealthiest? Take your pick: it could be the high-protein/high-fat diet or the low-protein/low-fat diet. They all wreak havoc on your waistline *and* your cardiovascular health.

It is easy to understand how all this happens. We live in an on-the-go culture, and twelve-hour workdays are not uncommon. Women who stay at home with their small children are caught in a similar time crunch.

Our fast-paced lifestyle also contributes to great mental stress and emotional isolation. Tragically, social ties are not as valued in our culture as they are in others. In many parts of the world, family comes first, and job comes second. In our culture, we work first and play later, if (and when) we have the time.

If family and friends are way down on our list of priorities, spirituality comes dead last. Ignore your spiritual life at your physical peril. Studies show, however, that individuals with a strong faith tend to stay healthier and live longer.[10] No matter which religion or approach to spirituality they choose, these women and men certainly are happier.

How Menopause Affects Heart Health

Menopause may increase a woman's risk of heart disease. One study involved 76 untreated hypertensive premenopausal women, 76 postmenopausal women, 30 normotensive premenopausal women, and 30 postmenopausal women who were matched for age, blood pressure, body mass index (BMI), and smoking. Researchers found that the degree to which blood pressure fell from day to night was less in both normotensive and hypertensive postmenopausal women than premenopausal women.[11]

This study and other similar ones point out that female hormones play a role in the health of all organs, and that increasing age may increase certain risk factors for the development of cardiovascular disease. Menopause appears to be associated with early structural and functional manifestations of heart disease, independent of age, obesity, blood pressure, and other confounding factors.

Goals for This Book

If you are a woman, or if you care about women, this book is for you. Discovering the various issues that increase the risk of a cardiovascular event may help you (or them) take the steps needed to prevent the event. Consider the adage, "Forewarned is fore armed." If we know what we're facing, we can face it square on and solve it.

As a clinical nutritionist, one of Carol's greatest joys is presenting factual information to her clients or students, seeing them make lifestyle and dietary changes, and rejoicing with them as their health improves. Even if heart disease "runs in your family," it is likely that you can avoid dying from a heart condition if you start making these changes early enough. That is good news.

In *A Woman's Guide to a Healthy Heart*, we hope to help women recognize how their emotions are inextricably intertwined with their cardiovascular health. The emotional lives of women and men are not exactly the same. A woman's emotions are a double-edged sword: they can increase the risk of heart disease, or they can help build a stronger heart. When a woman has a heart event or stroke, her emotions can delay recovery or facilitate recovery. Emotions are a powerful tool, for both destruction and healing.

Certainly, however, emotions are not the only factor in heart health. We will also address the importance of diet. There is a huge amount of confusion in the marketplace over the question, "What is a healthy diet?" We'll sort through all the ambiguities and conflicting information and make it simple to construct a heart-healthy, brain-healthy diet. We'll learn why it is important to avoid smoking, excess drinking, and other harmful lifestyle practices. We'll discuss supplements: which ones support heart health and other related systems. We'll even address the nagging issue of exercise! Yes, you know you should, but why? And how? Taking care of your emotional health is critical, but you can do so much to improve your health through lifestyle and live to a ripe old age.

Heart disease is a complex illness, and a "magic bullet," or a cure-all, doesn't exist. The medical community is finally recognizing that we need to attend to every aspect of our lives in order to promote healthy hearts.

Achieving a healthy emotional life may yield some unexpected benefits. When a woman cares about herself and her life, she is likely to feel more motivated to eat better, work out regularly, quit smoking, and do whatever it takes to get healthy and stay that way.

Above all, this book will help you take responsibility for your own good health.

CHAPTER 1

The Heart of a Woman and How It Works

W E KNOW OUR HEARTS WORK HARD. How could they not? Just imagine working every minute of your life for more than seventy-five years without even a moment to rest.

But how exactly does your heart work? What does it look like? What does it require for optimum functioning? How can we support its efforts?

The human heart is a pump about the size of a human fist, and nestles in the center of the chest just under the rib cage, protected from exterior trauma. Each of its four chambers is actively involved in oxygenating the blood as it flows through the body; this is the prime task of the pumping mechanism (see Figure 1.1). After the blood shuttles oxygen to every cell of the body, it flows back from the veins, depleted of oxygen, into the upper chamber on the right side of the heart (the right atrium). It then drops into the lower chamber (the right ventricle).

From the right ventricle, the blood is pumped through the pulmonary artery into the lungs. The hemoglobin in the blood gathers up oxygen; then the blood moves from the lungs through the pulmonary veins and flows into the upper chamber on the left side of the heart (the left atrium).

From there, the oxygen-rich blood drops into the lower chamber (left ventricle), and is pumped out to the body through the aorta, its largest artery. Through a complex system of arteries, veins, and capillaries, blood carries oxygen and nutrients to every part of the body. At the same time, it sweeps away waste materials generated by the cells and brings them to the liver for transport out of the body.

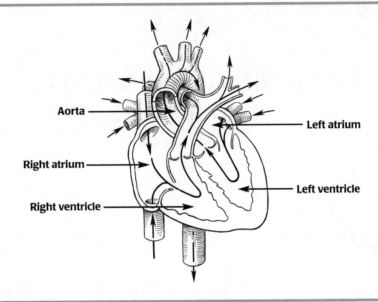

Figure 1.1 Cutaway view of the human heart showing the four chambers actively involved in oxygenating blood as it flows through the body.

WHEN THE HEART DOESN'T WORK RIGHT

How does the heart break down? In what different forms does heart disease manifest itself? First, let's look at some of the primary forms of heart disease and some additional heart-related terms.

- **Angina** is a chest pain that happens when the heart isn't getting the blood supply it needs during periods of high demand, such as strenuous exercise or excitement. In a healthy cardiovascular system, the coronary arteries widen so they can send more blood to the heart.
- **Arrhythmia** is an irregular heartbeat. The underlying heart disease that causes the arrhythmia offers more reason for concern than the arrhythmia itself. Arrhythmias may cause dizziness, light-headedness, and fainting.
- **Atherosclerosis,** or "hardening of the arteries," can be blamed on high blood pressure. When blood pressure gets too high, it creates tiny cracks in the inner walls of the arteries. These cracks make it perilously easy for fatty deposits to build up, thereby narrowing the arteries. As a result of this buildup, the arteries stiffen, cannot expand, and are unable to send as much blood as the heart demands.

- **Bacterial endocarditis** refers to inflammation of the smooth arterial lining of the heart (endocardium). Gingivitis, skin infections, and other infections in the body may release bacteria into the bloodstream, thereby causing endocarditis.
- **Cardiomyopathy** refers to any disease of the heart muscle. It changes the structure or damages the function of the wall of the ventricles (the lower chambers of the heart). It is a progressive disorder and often stems from coronary arterary disease.
- **Congestive heart failure** occurs when the heart doesn't pump enough blood to meet the body's needs for oxygen and nutrients.
- **Echocardiogram,** a diagnostic test, employs an ultrasound probe with sound waves to generate pictures of the heart. An echocardiogram reveals the shape, texture, and motion of the valves. It also assesses heart function and the size of the heart muscle and its chambers.
- **Endothelium** is the lining of an artery wall. The endothelium helps regulate artery function, such as dilation and contraction.
- **Heart attack,** also known as a myocardial infarction, occurs when the blood supply is drastically decreased or stopped. It can cause sudden death.
- **High blood pressure** can lead to heart disease and stroke. Blood pressure refers to the force of the blood traveling through the arteries. It is measured by counting the number of times the heart contracts (systolic), and the rests between the heartbeats (diastolic). Normal blood pressure is 120/80.
- **Ischemic** comes from two Greek words meaning *keeping back* and *blood*. Ischemic heart disease refers to the obstruction of blood flow. Atherosclerosis is the most common obstruction. This is due to a buildup of fats and calcium on the inner walls of the coronary arteries.
- **Mitral valve prolapse** occurs when the valve leaflets expand into the left atrium while the ventricles are contracting. As a result, small amounts of blood may leak into the atrium. A mitral valve prolapse rarely produces symptoms and does not usually lead to serious heart problems.
- **Peripheral vascular disease** is a disease of the circulatory system. It is a narrowing of the blood vessels in the arms and legs. Cigarette smoking and diabetes are two suspected culprits in the disease. It is more common in men than in women.
- **Stroke** falls into at least two categories: ischemic stroke and brain hemorrhage. An ischemic stroke occurs when the blood flow to the brain is blocked. When a blood vessel in the brain ruptures, brain hemorrhage occurs. Both types of stroke lead to the death of brain cells and brain tissues. As a result, the components of the body that those cells regulated may not function. Stroke can cause partial paralysis; loss of speech, memory, or understanding; or death.

The human heart never takes a break. It pumps whether you're awake or asleep. The average heart beats approximately 100,000 times a day, pumping about 1,800 gallons of blood.

Is Heart Disease a Woman's Issue?

Heart disease as a woman's issue kind of "sneaked up" on us, just as it must have "sneaked up" on men around the turn of the twentieth century. Before that time, heart disease was extremely rare, and many doctors never treated a cardiovascular patient in their professional lives.

Stressors mounted, however, as the twentieth century became more technology driven. Men (and women) moved from the quiet peace of farms into the bustling, noisy cities to take jobs in factories and offices. They lost a great deal of control over their lives, a major stress inducer.

As they moved from the farms, they forfeited the fresh food they raised themselves, and technology took over here as well. The food didn't taste good as it bounced off the assembly line, so producers added thousands of chemicals to make their food look like it was farm fresh; indeed, it often tasted better than the farm-raised stuff because of flavor enhancers. Slowly, people were lured away from the natural food provided since the dawn of time into a pseudofood culture that left the body bereft of the nutrition it needed for vibrant health.

The Crazy Makers: How the Food Industry Is Destroying Our Brains and Harming Our Children, by Carol Simontacchi (Tarcher/Putnam, 2000), explores how the modern food culture is affecting the structure and function of the human brain. It is a terrifying look at what is going wrong with our mental health and how pseudofood is contributing to the breakdown of the human brain. In this

RED BLOOD CELLS

The work of the red blood cell (RBC) truly is astonishing! More than 90 percent of the formed elements in the blood are erythrocytes, or red blood cells containing hemoglobin, onto which oxygen is piggybacked. Each RBC contains about 280 million hemoglobin molecules; all their internal space is used for oxygen transport. Yet as active as the RBCs are, both synthesizing and using ATP (adenosine triphosphate or cellular energy), they do not use any of their transport oxygen in the production of energy. Amazing!

book, we will see that the food culture is destroying our hearts as well. We simply aren't eating what our hearts need to be healthy and strong for a lifetime.

So, as the twentieth century raced toward the twenty-first, and the pace of life increased even more, women began falling prey to heart disease, just like their husbands.

There were (and still are) some differences in heart disease for men and women, however. Researchers were still looking at heart disease as a "man's illness" and decided not to include women in their studies on it. They neglected to realize that while heart disease strikes men and women with about equal frequency, the manifestation of the disease could be profoundly different.

As a result, science is just now catching up to the idea that if doctors are going to prevent heart disease in their female patients, they are going to have to learn about how women experience this illness. Fortunately, science is catching on—we just had to wait a few more decades, and a few more women had to die before the research caught up.

Is There a History of Gender Bias in Medicine?

One might suspect that the bias in health care reflects the underlying values in Western culture. Do individuals deemed most important in society receive the highest quality of care? It's an unsettling question with no clear answer.[1]

Both men and women need to be informed about heart disease; it is an issue for both genders. However, the illness may be more important for women, considering the medical bias they have experienced over the years. We just haven't received the medical attention we need to maintain the health of our hearts.

Throughout history, women have often been regarded—consciously or unconsciously—as "walking wombs." Iris Litt, M.D., author of *Taking Our Pulse: The Health of America's Women* (Stanford University Press, 1997), noted that her father, also a doctor, believed that women's health problems could all be attributed to the menstrual cycle.[2]

When the American Medical Association met in 1893, one lecturer claimed that the five leading causes of illness in women were incomplete development of the sex organs; gonorrhea; septic inflammation after childbirth; rough tears in the flesh caused by childbirth; and other factors, including constipation, poor lifestyle choices, and "errors of dress."

The possibility of heart disease in women was typically ignored, even though since at least 1908, heart disease has been the leading cause of death in American women. The American Heart Association sponsored its first conference on women and heart disease in 1964—fifty-six years later. To add insult to injury, the conference did not address women's heart health; it discussed how women could protect their husbands from heart disease.[3]

The Unique Medical Struggles of African American Women

To this day, African American women face a double whammy: gender and race. In the early twentieth century, many educated white Southerners still believed that African Americans were physically and psychologically unfit for freedom, explains Edward H. Beardsley in *Women, Health, and Medicine in America*, edited by Rima D Apple (Rutgers University Press, 1990). They believed that African American women and men faced certain extinction. Therefore, they reasoned, public health and medical efforts to aid African Americans were a waste of precious resources.

Eventually, it became clear that African Americans were not dying out, and, in fact, were multiplying. Black women may have been denied good maternal and obstetrical care because, unconsciously perhaps, white male physicians feared the possibility that blacks would eventually outnumber whites.

By 1900, heart and kidney disease were the leading causes of death in African American women and men. Whites, too, had a high death rate from cardiovascular disease, but black women died four times more often than did white women.

There were other reasons for this medical disparity. In the early 1900s, about 75 percent of African Americans lived in the South. They were typically poor and could not afford food or medical care. A lack of education and literacy made it difficult for black women to learn how to protect their own health.[4]

These factors have improved, but we have a long way to go to achieve racial equality. An article in the *Harvard Public Health Review* notes that African Americans are poor in disproportionate numbers. People who live in poverty are more likely to be exposed to lead paint, or to live close to chemical plants and waste incinerators. The poor often eat high-fat and high-salt food, rather than fruits or vegetables. Besides personal choice, this may be due to the increasing scarcity of affordable, inner-city grocery stores. Furthermore, the pressures of poverty lead to higher rates of smoking and alcohol abuse.[5]

Lack of health insurance is another contributing factor to the inequity of health care. Almost 23 percent of African American women and men have no health insurance. Many of these individuals work full-time at low-paying jobs that don't provide insurance benefits. The Kaiser report confirms that almost 40 percent of the uninsured delay seeing the doctor. Thirty percent don't fill their prescriptions.[6]

Disrespect Is Dangerous for Women

We have seen in the research that it takes women longer to get to the emergency room when they believe they are experiencing a heart attack, and longer for them to be admitted to the cardiovascular unit in the hospital once the diagnosis has been made.

One of the reasons for this disparity appears to be that women are, by nature, caregivers more than care receivers. They tend to take care of the family before themselves and may be unaccustomed to asking for help when they need it. Women will often sacrifice their own needs on the altar of their husband's or children's demands.

Another real possibility, however, is that women are so accustomed to being told "It's all in your head," or "You are just depressed, honey" that they don't think they'll be believed when they do get to the hospital. When that first sign of heart disease presents, imagine what happens in her mind, "It probably is all in my head . . . I'm just tired today . . . I'm a little down today. I don't want to bother the doctor or my husband . . ." We've just gotten used to the condecension. We don't respect our own intuition because no one else does, either.

We simply must get beyond this "learned helplessness" to a position of internal and external power. We must take charge of our health.

How can we confront this professional apathy or ignorance in the doctor's office? We must become informed consumers of medical care. One of the best ways to take charge of one's health is to select a physician who approaches health care from a holistic model. A holistic model of health takes into consideration the entire body, not just an organ or a system. A holistic physician is trained in nutrition and uses food as part of the healing process.

A holistic physician will ask questions about diet, exercise, stress, lifestyle, and symptoms. He or she will take a partnership role, not a dominating one, in discussions about diagnoses, treatment, and health management. Carol simply refuses to work with a doctor who does not involve her in an intelligent conversation about her needs, and who will not expect her or allow her to become involved in her healing process.

If Carol must use a certain physician because of insurance demands, she uses the physician for a diagnosis, then takes the diagnosis to a physician who understands holistic healing. Together they work on her health needs. In other words, she hires her physician to take care of her specific needs. She does not simply acquiesce. (Yes, she's probably considered to be "noncompliant" or a "difficult patient!")

The (Scary) History of Heart Research for Women

Typically, women have been excluded from drug studies, even though they use more medications and medical services than do men. Researchers have claimed that this neglect was benign and inadvertent.[7] One reason may be that the research community was populated with men; female researchers were few and not, for the most part, in positions of authority.

After the U.S. military found evidence of atrocious medical experiments at the Nazi concentration camps, the nation took a more protective approach to medical research. Pregnant women, or any woman of childbearing age, were considered a vulnerable population. The argument was that drug tests in women in their childbearing years might affect fertility or the health of the fetus.

Some of this protectiveness was a reaction to the thalidomide debacle in the 1950s. Pregnant mothers took this drug to reduce nausea, and the result was thousands of deformed children. None of us "older women" can forget the images of deformed babies that flooded the media during this horrible period of medical history. Understandably, researchers are reluctant to expose women to experimental drugs during their childbearing years.

Although this argument certainly has merit, the majority of women afflicted with heart disease are past their childbearing years. Furthermore, many new medications are insufficiently studied for women, even though female hormones are a major influence on the genesis and progression of the disease.[8]

It was the "little issue" of hormones that slanted the research toward males, however. Researchers feared that hormonal shifts could complicate their work. They would have to increase their sample size, which would cost both time and money. They would have to write new study protocols that took into account the hormonal variable.

Instead of gearing 50 percent of the research toward the other 50 percent of the population, they took the simple route and just excluded women, extrapolating the data finds to females. This practice clearly violates the scientific method and invalidates much of the research findings for women.

In addition, during the first half of the twentieth century, many studies recruited medical students, who were typically men.[9]

Here are further examples of the "ol' boys' club" in medical research:

- No women were included in the widely quoted and highly respected 1982 Multiple Risk Factor Intervention Trial (MRFIT). Its focus was to assess the impact of lifestyle factors on cholesterol levels and heart disease—in men.[10]
- No women were included in a Harvard School of Public Health study on the impact of caffeine on heart disease.[11]
- No women were included in the first twenty years of the Baltimore Longitudinal Study, one of the largest studies undertaken on the aging process. (Gene Cohen, then deputy director of the National Institute on Aging, explained that only one toilet was available in its facility.)
- Astonishingly, no women were included in a pilot project at Rockefeller University—in order to learn about how obesity affected breast and uterine cancer, researchers used men. Senator Olympia Snowe commented (tongue in cheek), "Somehow, I find it hard to believe that the male-dominated medical community would tolerate a study of prostate cancer that used only women as research subjects."[12]

Is there a vast, tightly organized secret male conspiracy at work? It's not likely. Florence Haseltine, M.D., of the National Institutes of Health, states, "I don't think [the bias] was malicious or intentional. You want doctors to study what they're interested in, so you have male doctors in their fifties studying other male doctors in their fifties for heart attacks. It's like everything else in our society. Women are second-class citizens, so they are thought of second."

Why Does It Matter?

Gender bias in medical research isn't just an academic issue. Women are *not* merely smaller versions of men, and they may experience disease and treatments very differently than men do. Consider the following examples:

- For decades, postmenopausal women with cholesterol higher than 200 have been urged to lower it. Of course, this recommendation is based on cholesterol studies on men. Although 200 and less is considered an ideal cholesterol level for a man, it may be different for women. Recent research indicates that the rate of heart attacks in women with 295-plus cholesterol levels is the same or lower than in men with cholesterol levels of 204.[13]
- Medications have different effects on women than on men. Most drug studies exclude women, however.
- Women may process medications differently than men do, because of hormonal fluctuations.

The result? Many doctors prescribe medications to women that have been insufficiently studied for them. These doctors don't necessarily know whether the drugs work for women, or whether the dosage they prescribed is safe. They don't consider whether doses should be modified according to the phases of the menstrual cycle.

Present-Day Bias in Treatment

Unfortunately, women of all races and ethnic backgrounds still face gender and racial bias as health care consumers. One study investigated the influence of gender, as well as race, on physicians' recommendations for chest pain. Eight actors, playing the role of patients, gave doctors a scripted description of their symptoms. The actors dressed identically, reported identical insurance and jobs, and acted identically during their interviews with doctors. The only variables in these "patients" were gender, race, and age.

The doctors were asked to assess their patients' chest pain, and to decide whether they wanted to refer their patients for tests. After the doctors were shown the results of their patients' stress tests, they were asked if they wanted to recommend cardiac catheterization for their patients.

The physicians involved understood that they were being surveyed on their diagnosis of chest pain, but they were unaware that the researchers were studying their responses based on gender and race. The authors of this study used multimedia presentations of interviews of patients who reported chest pains.

The results indicated that men and Caucasians were more likely to be referred for cardiac catheterization than women and African Americans. Authors David Benjamin Oppenheimer and Marjorie M. Schultz write, "[This] study provides evidence of race and gender stereotyping that is likely not intentional, but that does produce racially and sexually disparate treatment."

The study also explored physicians' assessment of the actor-patients' personalities. The physicians judged the female patients as being less intelligent, less self-controlled, and more inclined to overreport symptoms than the male patients. When comparing white male patients with black female patients, physicians judged white men as friendlier, smarter, more self-controlled, more independent, more communicative, and more content.

Furthermore, the study suggests that part of this apparent bias is due to differences in insurance coverage, lack of access to health care, disparate socioeconomic levels, noncompliant patients, and economic barriers.

Oppenheimer and Schultz conclude,

> Essential also is a recognition that precisely because the problem is unconscious, rectification necessarily involves developing new awareness that stereotypes do affect judgments and perceptions of even the most well-intentioned people. Elimination of biases requires vigorous retraining of judgments and perpetual vigilance.[14]

What does "retraining of judgments and perpetual vigilance" mean? We certainly cannot expect the male-dominated medical profession to take care of this for us. We women are going to have to "train" our physicians to stop thinking like a "male-dominated medical paradigm" and challenge their own personal biases.

How do we do that? By listening, questioning, evaluating, and prodding until we get the answers we need.

Want to excite a stimulating conversation among women? Start asking questions about what happened the last time they went to the doctor. You'll hear a litany of bad diagnoses and disrespect that is both insulting and dangerous. Wrong diagnoses and disrespect are particularly perilous when it comes to heart and cardiovascular diseases.

Today, gender bias in medical research continues. In one study focusing on 185,000 men and women in a London hospital, researchers found that men were more likely than women to receive treatment for blood clots, to be given secondary prevention through other medications, to undergo exercise testing and coronary angiography, and to undergo an echocardiogram.[15]

The old assumptions about hormone replacement therapy have also impeded adequate treatment for women. (See Chapter 3 for more details.)

Women in Medicine

The bias doesn't stop with female patient care. Female health care providers have faced an uphill battle, even though throughout the ages, healing has been more the domain of women than men.

Women hold an honored place in the history of medicine. Evidence suggests that women were treating patients and performing surgery at least three thousand years ago. In the early history of medicine, it was typically women who prepared herbal medicines, delivered babies, and gave daily care to the sick.

Fortunately, today, despite many setbacks over the centuries in the field of medicine, women comprise 40 percent of medical school students. (In contrast, in 1970, only 13 percent of medical students were women.) An estimated 18 percent of practicing physicians are women. It hasn't been easy: female physicians face a dearth of mentors, an environment of exclusion, unequal salary, sexual harassment, the problems of balancing a demanding profession and parenthood, and even battles over lab space.

In one sense, although participation in the medical community is a positive step for women, it hasn't necessarily changed the medical paradigm. Female doctors can be just as insensitive to the special needs of women as their male counterparts, probably because they are educated and trained in a male model of medicine. While women tend to be more holistic in their thinking, the western medical model is still a reductionistic one: reducing the body to its individual parts and treating the parts instead of the system or the organism. Women doctors are just as likely as male physicians to elevate the scientific method to the level of godhood, to disregard the traditions of the ancients, and to "think like a man" instead of thinking like a healer.

Perhaps the best thing that could happen to the medical profession, in terms of female health, would be to train female doctors in a holistic model instead of the twentieth-century medical model.

The Future Looks Promising

Gender equity in medicine is progressing, albeit slowly. In 1989, an audit of NIH research showed that less than one in seven dollars was used for women's health research. The report on this discrepancy also noted that women were underrepresented in medical research. The result was the creation of the Office of Research on Women's Health in 1990.

The National Institutes of Health launched the Women's Health Initiative (WHI) in 1991. The focus of the WHI is to protect against the most common causes of death, disability, and decreased quality of life in postmenopausal women. The WHI has investigated potential benefits and risks linked with hormone replacement therapy, dietary supplements, and other factors that may help prevent heart disease and other serious illnesses.

The Office of Research on Women's Health (ORWH) is supporting a report titled "Understanding the Biology of Sex and Gender Differences." In this study, researchers will review and explain medicine's current level of knowledge and make recommendations for filling in the research gaps.

Even the government is finally acknowledging the gender bias found in medicine. The Government Accounting Office accused the National Institutes of Health of "excluding women from most studies involving diseases, treatments, and drug effects, and for devoting only 13 percent of its research funds for women."

To promote gender equity in medicine, author Catherine Heath suggests that medical schools expose their students to a more realistic picture of patient populations. She also recommends that research not concerning gender-specific issues (for example, prostate and uterine cancer) include both men and women. Furthermore, she recommends that we support lobbying for gender- unbiased research funding, which could lead to more accurate research results. Finally, Heath urges women to become informed patients and to assert themselves to doctors who ignore their concerns.[16]

Clearly, gender and racial bias in medicine reflects the gender and racial bias in our society. Greater equality in medicine will only occur when we achieve greater equality on a cultural level. This problem needs to be addressed on all fronts: medical, political, professional, and personal. It's an ongoing struggle that every woman and ethnic minority have to face.

Mary Harper, Ph.D., states,

> As we enter an increasingly global society, women's health advocates and activists worldwide will need to confront how culture, living, and working conditions, not just medical care, actually produce health . . . we need to acknowledge the degree to which the future of women's health worldwide lies not just in medical care, but in gender equity and social justice.[17]

CHAPTER 2

How Women
Experience Heart Disease

OF WHICH DISEASES ARE WOMEN MOST AFRAID? Cancer? Stroke? Dementia? Heart disease? If we look at what health conditions concern women most, we're looking at weight (number one) and age-related dementia (number two). We don't want to get fat and we don't want to lose our minds.

When it comes to the question, "What do most women die from?" and therefore, "what am I more likely to die from?" we're looking at breast cancer. We also fear other forms of cancer, Alzheimer's disease, and accidents, but we should be looking at heart disease. Cardiovascular disease, in all its forms and permutations, kills far more women than all types of cancer combined.

The facts on women and heart disease are sobering. The American Heart Association reports that:

- Cardiovascular disease (CVD) accounts for 43.3 percent of all female deaths in the United States and most developed countries.
- CVD caused the deaths of 502,938 females in 1997. In contrast, all forms of cancer caused the deaths of 258,467 women.
- Thirty-eight percent of women will die within a year after having a heart attack. Conversely, only 25 percent of men will die within a year of experiencing a heart event.
- Meanwhile, the myth still prevails that CVD is not a genuine threat to women.[1]

Heart Disease Is Number One

So far the message hasn't gotten through to women that they need to take care of their hearts, and that they need to watch for the ominous signs of an impending heart attack. Yet coronary heart disease is responsible for one out of every two deaths among women.

The good news about the rate of heart disease is that it has been declining over the past several years. It is declining more rapidly for men than for women, however.

The misperception that heart attacks primarily affect overweight, middle-aged, harried businessmen is not just a mental block (or ignorance) in the minds of the lay public. The medical establishment sometimes forgets that heart disease ends the lives of women prematurely, and this medical blind spot has cut short the lives of many women.

One study claims that within the first month after a heart attack, the death rate for women is more than double the death rate of men.[2] The research included more than 1,400 people under the age of eighty who had had a first heart attack. The study included 331 women and 1,129 men. Researchers reported that the death rate for women was 18.5 percent, whereas for men, it was only 8.3 percent.[3] Why the disparity in death rates for men and women?

Dr. Nanette Wenger from the Emory University School of Medicine pointed out study flaws. Other factors, however, point to huge disparities in the diagnosis and treatment that women receive when they present their symptoms to the emergency room or doctor:

1. The women in this study were older than the men.
2. The women were more likely to suffer from diabetes and other related illnesses.
3. The men received more intense care than the women did.
4. The men received better follow-up care than the women did.
5. The men were typically referred earlier for balloon angioplasty or bypass surgery than the women were.
6. The women didn't appear to understand that they were susceptible to heart attacks.[4]

Diabetes is a major risk factor for the development of cardiovascular illness. Because diabetes occurs more frequently in women than men, women are more likely to succumb to heart disease. The ages of the women in the study were significantly higher than the men. How would the statistics have appeared if the researchers had leveled the ages in the statistical equation, or had included equal numbers of men and women? Perhaps the results would have been different.

But the researchers noted that men generally received better medical care than women, and that *women were oblivious to the fact that they could be susceptible to heart disease.* They just didn't know they had a potential problem.

Fortunately for women, their heart attacks generally occur about seven or eight years later than in men. Most men become vulnerable to heart disease between the ages of forty-five and fifty-five. In contrast, women don't usually experience heart trouble until after menopause. In the United States, the average age of menopause is fifty-one. Unfortunately for women, if they do have a heart attack between ages forty-five and fifty-five, they have a greater risk of dying.[5]

Diagnosis of heart disease in women still lags behind diagnosis in men. However, it appears that one diagnostic technique, the contrast echocardiography, is particularly effective in women. Echocardiography measures ultrasound waves. This method is often used when a mitral valve prolapse or other valvular problems are suspected.

What Does a Female Heart Attack Look Like?

We commonly associate a heart attack with a sudden squeezing in the chest and pain throughout the left arm. When confronted with that symptom, most people realize they may be having a heart attack and seek immediate help. Symptoms vary from person to person, though. Other symptoms may present in the absence of chest squeezing or arm pain, and some people do not even realize they have had, or are having, a heart attack.

What are other common symptoms? Sometimes a heart attack generates subtle signs: a mild chest discomfort or a dull ache in the chest, or heart palpitations, nausea, vomiting, weakness, dizziness, coughing, fainting, and cold perspiration. Other symptoms may include a tingling sensation in the hands, wrists, and fingers; pain in the shoulders, neck, and jaw; pain in the teeth and back; indigestion; and dry mouth.

Sometimes there is no pain at all—the chest pain we typically associate with a heart attack does not always occur. These are called "silent heart attacks." Elderly men and women and people with diabetes face the highest risk of a silent heart attack.

Symptoms in Women

Although many symptoms overlap, women frequently have more atypical symptoms of heart attack than men do. Their symptoms may be more obtuse, or might be attributed to other health problems. Women are more likely to experience shortness of breath or excessive sweating. They may feel intense fatigue or nausea; they may simply "intuitively believe" they are having a heart attack in the absence of other clearly defined complaints. Sadly, doctors and nurses often misdiagnose these as menopausal symptoms or other health conditions. Instead of submitting women to a diagnostic evaluation that could point the finger at heart disease, they send them home with a prescription for an antidepressant or some other medication designed to relieve their anxiety. They dismiss women's complaints, and as a result, many women die unnecessarily.

Angina pectoris—characterized by chest pain—does occur in women. Even so, women are more likely to delay treatment. Even when women suspect that this symptom is related to heart disease, they may feel compelled to "self-treat to maintain control."[6] Of course, this delay may well result in extensive heart damage and premature death. As noted previously, it takes women about one hour longer to present to the emergency room of the hospital when they feel or experience their first symptoms than it does for men. That hour can mean the difference between life or death, between comparatively little damage to the heart muscle and massive injury that could have been prevented.

Women aren't the only ones who fail to consider heart disease as a potential cause of their discomfort. Sometimes medical personnel delay treatment. There may be several reasons for this medical oversight. Women are slightly less likely than men to exhibit familiar EKG findings. Their symptoms are not as easily "read"; they may be more inconclusive at first glance. Heart disease is more commonly associated with men than women, so "heart attack" may not be the first thought in the practitioner's mind when he or she is confronted with a less obvious symptom profile. As a result, doctors delay admitting women to the cardiovascular unit of the hospital by an hour or more.

Once they are admitted for further evaluation, women still may not receive equal treatment. Although women with heart attacks are often much more ill than men, they are less likely to get aggressive clot-busting medications. Even after discharge, women are less likely than men to be scheduled for cardiac rehabilitation or exercise testing.[7]

More Women Die

Although their premenopausal risk for heart disease may be lower, women are more vulnerable to *fatal* heart attacks. A *Mayo Clinic Health Letter* shares some factors that may account for this disparity:

- *Age.* Older women may not be robust enough to survive a heart attack, or to endure angioplasty, surgery, or other common treatments.
- *Misdiagnosis.* Because women are more likely to report unusual symptoms of heart attack, the problem may not be recognized. Lack of treatment leads to more—and often fatal—damage to the heart.
- *Ignorance.* Many women delay medical treatment because they're less likely than men to think they're having a heart attack. Women who think that heart attacks just don't happen to women may ignore important symptoms. When they finally do present themselves to a doctor, the damage may be extensive and more challenging to treat. Some women who suffer from a heart attack have no symptoms at all—until they die.
- *Size.* In years past, it was believed that women's smaller hearts and blood vessels made them more difficult to treat. However, Mayo Clinic doctors now assert that the seriousness of the heart disease is a more significant factor than gender differences or variations in the size of the organ.
- *Diabetes.* Coronary artery disease and heart-related fatalities are more likely to occur in women with diabetes than in men with diabetes. Women with diabetes are twice as likely to experience a second heart attack than their male counterparts.[8]

REGION AND RACE MAKE A DIFFERENCE

Death rates from heart disease not only vary among races, they also vary among regions throughout the United States. The Center for Disease Control and Prevention (CDC) and West Virginia University (WVU) have created an unusual atlas: *Women and Heart Disease: An Atlas of Racial and Ethnic Disparities in Mortality*. More than two hundred national and state maps were used to identify heart disease deaths among women for the years 1991–1995. Among its findings are the following facts:

Overall, the highest heart disease death rates among women were found in parts of the rural South, including the Mississippi Delta and Appalachian regions. In contrast, the lowest heart disease death rates for women occur in counties in the Pacific Northwest, the Rocky Mountain areas of Colorado and New Mexico, and parts of Wisconsin, North Dakota, and South Dakota.

Why do differences occur among regions and ethnic populations? The authors of this atlas noted underlying factors such as economic resources, the social isolation of older women, and the availability of medical facilities.[9]

More information about this atlas is available online at www.cdc.gov/nccdphp /cvd/womensatlas.

Women and Strokes

Stroke is another form of heart disease that needs to be brought into the cardiovascular disease discussion. Every year, stroke kills 160,000 Americans. Stroke is the third leading cause of death in this country and the leading cause of disability. Twenty-five percent of strokes strike people under the age of sixty-five. Of the four million stroke victims who survive, two-thirds suffer from moderate to severe disabilities.

Consider the following statistics on strokes and women, from the National Stroke Association:

- About 100,000 young and middle-aged women suffer from strokes every year.
- African American women are at highest risk of stroke.
- Although women account for only 43 percent of strokes, they account for 61 percent of stroke deaths.

In a small number of people, heart surgery triggers strokes. In women, that risk is 21 percent higher than in men. Women who suffer stroke are more likely than men to die from the event. Dr. Victor G. Davila-Roman, M.D., one of the authors of an analysis of stroke risk, noted that just being a woman is "an independent risk factor for stroke even after we adjusted for known stroke risks." Stroke risk factors include diabetes, age, smoking, high cholesterol, and high blood pressure.

Dr. Davila-Roman noted that, in this particular analysis, 3.8 percent of stroke victims were women, and only 2.4 percent were men. Within a month after the surgery, the death rate for women was 5.7 percent. In contrast, only 3.5 percent of the men died.[10]

Factors Contributing to Stroke

What makes women more vulnerable to fatal strokes than men? First of all, high blood pressure affects 29 million American women, and more than 50 percent of women over age fifty-five. According to the National Institute

---

STROKE SYMPTOMS

Common symptoms of stroke among women and men include:

- Face, arm, or leg becomes numb or weak, particularly on one side of the body.
- Sudden confusion, or difficulty with speaking or understanding.
- Sudden difficulty in seeing with one or both eyes.
- Sudden dizziness, loss of balance and coordination, and difficulty in walking.
- Sudden excruciating headache, with no known cause.
- Sudden change in personality or mental acuity, or sudden memory loss.

Strokes—among both women and men—exact a steep price in mortality, morbidity, and expense. According to the National Stroke Association, strokes cost our country approximately $43 billion a year. Twenty-eight billion dollars a year is spent on medical care and therapy.[11]

of Neurological Disorders and Strokes, an individual is four to six times more likely to experience a stroke if she or he has hypertension.[12]

What causes high blood pressure? Again, we think of hypertension as being a "man's disease" brought on by the pressures of life, accompanied by unhealthy indulgences.

Perhaps those same factors contribute to hypertension in women. As we have seen, women are struggling with an equal (or perhaps greater) amount of stress than their male counterparts. They, too, are caught in time pressures that make it difficult for them to care for themselves. We will see in a later chapter how each of these factors contributes to heart disease. They contribute to hypertension as well. Of course, hypertension is a precursor to stroke and other forms of cardiovascular disease.

A healthy blood pressure for women aged eighteen and older is lower than 130/85 millimeters of mercury (mmHg), according to the National Heart, Lung, and Blood Institute (NHLBI). A high/normal blood pressure—130/85 to 139/89—is enough to raise your risk of the following conditions: stroke, kidney problems, blindness, and atherosclerosis ("hardening of the arteries").

High blood pressure produces no symptoms. But while it is silent, it is not benign. Imperceptibly, the health of the organs is being compromised. Only when severe damage has occurred to the kidneys or cardiovascular system do symptoms appear, often in the form of a fatal heart attack or stroke.

The National Institutes of Health recommends blood pressure checks at least once every two years. If your blood pressure is higher than 130/85, ask your physician about checking it more frequently. A blood pressure of 140/90 or higher, on three or more checkups, indicates hypertension and needs to be treated.[13]

The second risk factor is diabetes, the third leading cause of death in this country. Diabetes occurs more often in women than in men. After age forty-five, about twice as many women develop Type 2 (adult-onset) diabetes as do men. Diabetes makes it difficult to move sugar out of the bloodstream and into the cells, and blood clots can easily form with sugar in the blood. (We will discuss Syndrome X and insulin resistance in Chapter 3.)

Why would women suffer from diabetes at higher rates than men? We don't have all the answers to that question, but we do know that women are often "sugarholics." In other words, they eat huge amounts of sugar, processed carbohydrates, and processed fats, each of which increase insulin secretion and thus the risk of adult-onset diabetes. We are currently seeing huge increases in adult onset diabetes in *children*, a particularly ominous sign that serious health problems lie further down the road for the younger members of our society in the form of obesity, diabetes, hypertension, and heart disease.

Third, migraine headaches affect stroke risk, and most of the migraine sufferers in the U.S. are women. This severe type of headache may raise a woman's risk for stroke three to six times. If a woman has migraines, smokes, and takes oral contraceptives, she is thirty-four times more likely to experience a stroke.

Fourth, pregnancy is believed to increase the risk of stroke in vulnerable women. Pregnancy often leads to higher blood pressure, greater production of blood-clotting factors, considerable blood loss during delivery, more stress on the heart, and increased blood volume in the second and third trimesters.

Since strokes and heart disease usually occur in older women, however, they only rarely occur during pregnancy. Keep in mind that certain symptoms of pregnancy may mirror the symptoms of cardiovascular problems, such as fatigue, shortness of breath, swelling in the arms and legs, and occasional palpitations.

Diagnostic techniques that use radioactive substances should be avoided during pregnancy, because of possible danger to the fetus. An echocardiography appears to be safe for pregnant women, though.

Fifth, menopause increases a woman's risk of stroke, related to her declining levels of natural estrogen. For decades, well-meaning doctors prescribed pharmaceutical estrogen to postmenopausal women to protect them from heart disease. In July of 2001, however, the American Heart Association changed its mind. The AHA advised doctors to stop telling their female patients that hormone replacement therapy (HRT) would reduce their heart attack risk. This turnabout was the result of the Women's Health Initiative (WHI), a long-term study mentioned earlier that suggested, in some cases, that HRT actually increased the risk of heart attack. The study was ended prematurely for this reason. (For more on HRT, see Chapter 3.)

Sixth, our love affair with dieting may set us up for an increased risk of heart disease, in the form of diet drugs. Phenylpropanolamine (PPA), an active ingredient in more than four-hundred diet drugs and cold medicines, has been linked to unexplained hemorrhagic strokes (bleeding in the brain) in young women and children. A Yale study showed that the number of people suffering from strokes when taking PPA was higher than the number of people suffering from strokes who were not taking it. Furthermore, the greatest incidence of PPA–related hemorrhagic stroke occurred in women.[14]

Seventh, oral contraceptives combined with high blood pressure and diabetes increase a woman's risk of stroke.

Finally, it appears that some women are willing—consciously or unconsciously—to die of embarrassment. Some women delay getting medical attention because they may be embarrassed if it turns out that the symptoms are "nothing."

What Happens After a Stroke?

Most strokes occur suddenly, develop quickly, and damage the brain within minutes. Occasionally, strokes worsen gradually, over anywhere from several hours to a day or two. Stroke can cause swelling of the brain, which damages brain tissue.

The aftereffects of a stroke can be devastating. Some stroke survivors cannot breathe, eat, or drink without help. Stroke by-products also include difficulty speaking and emotional and sexual problems. Approximately 25 percent of stroke survivors go through a major depression. In addition, stroke may disable a person's ability to control her emotions.

However, many stroke survivors retrieve all or most of their normal function. About 50 percent of stroke survivors with one-sided paralysis, and most of those with less severe symptoms, recover some function before they leave the hospital. Only 20 percent die in the hospital; most of those are elderly.[15]

Rehabilitation is critical for stroke survivors. The rehabilitation team includes a physiatrist—a doctor who specializes in physical medicine and rehabilitation. In addition, a physical therapist, occupational therapist, speech therapist, social worker, and psychologist may be involved. The purpose is to improve the individual's mobility, ability to take care of herself, and restoration of recreational and vocational interests.

Risk Factors for Women

This information about cardiovascular disease is frightening, isn't it? Perhaps for the first time in our lives, we feel vulnerable to a life-threatening illness that may strike without warning, like a California earthquake. We thought our "femaleness" protected us from this most devastating illness.

The good news is that, if we change our diets, our lifestyle, attitudes, and use true preventive medicine, we can, for the most part, avoid getting heart disease or stroke in the first place. Of course, the good news comes with a little stinger attached: We will have to change our diets. We will have to get off the couch and exercise. We will have to work on our emotional health. We'll need to deal with other issues, but we can do it. Remember that prevention is always the easiest, most affordable, and most painless approach to good health.

Which risk factors are more relevant for women than for men?

High Blood Pressure

Although we typically associate high blood pressure with stroke, it is also a risk factor for heart attack. We should get our blood pressure checked on a regular basis. If it is higher than it should be, we should take care of it. Fortunately, nature provides some excellent tools for lowering blood pressure.

Cholesterol

High-density lipoprotein (HDL) is considered to be the "good" cholesterol. Low-density lipoprotein (LDL), or very low density lipoprotein (VLDL) is considered to be the "bad cholesterol." (Lipoproteins are lipids encased in proteins to help move them through the watery medium of the blood. Although lipoproteins are not purely fats, they help distribute fats to the body's tissues through the blood and lymph systems.)

These terms can be misleading. All types of cholesterol serve a useful function in the body. What is more important than total cholesterol levels is the ratio between these different fractions. Low levels of HDL cholesterol indicate a greater risk for heart disease in women than in men, according to the 1999 consensus panel statement by the American Heart Association (AHA) and the American College of Cardiology. High levels of HDL are considered to be protective against stroke and heart attack. Between the ages of twenty and thirty-four, and after menopause, women typically have higher total cholesterol than men.[16]

For women, HDL levels lower than 35 mg/dL increase the risk of coronary heart disease, according to the National Cholesterol Education Program (NCEP) of the National Institutes of Health (NIH). The ideal HDL levels are 45 mg/dL or higher. HDL cholesterol levels over 60 mg/dL are even better. Instead of getting a total cholesterol count when having blood work done, men and women should ask for HDL and LDL numbers, and take steps to elevate the HDL fraction. Unfortunately, high LDL cholesterol shows no warning signs. Typically, the first symptoms are chest pain or heart attack.

An increased risk of abnormal cholesterol is found in women and men with hypothyroidism, some kidney diseases, and diabetes.

High Triglyercides

Triglycerides are the fat cells that cling to the hips and stomach, and increase the risk of insulin resistance and heart disease. Triglycerides nestling in the upper part of the body indicate a prime risk of heart disease.

When these same triglycerides float in increasing amounts through the bloodstream, another risk factor develops. High serum triglycerides stick to the arterial walls, clogging up the arteries and setting the stage for a heart attack.

Observational studies suggest that high triglyceride levels are a stronger predictor for coronary heart disease in women than in men. Yet there is still some confusion about the causal relationship between triglycerides and heart disease. High triglyceride levels typically coexist with obesity, diabetes, high blood pressure, and low HDL levels, each one of which is a distinct risk factor for heart disease in both women and men.[17]

The 1999 consensus panel recommended triglyceride levels below 150 mg/dL for women. How does one lower triglyceride levels? Going "natural" is the best route. Enjoying several meals a week of fresh seafood (grilled or baked), avocados, raw nuts and seeds, and moderate amounts of butter promotes healthy triglyceride and cholesterol levels. We needn't be afraid of fat *if* the fats are natural and are balanced with fresh fruits and vegetables that help clean excess fatty acids out of the body. A diet that is high in fiber helps normalize cholesterol and triglyceride levels. Of course, weight control; a low-fat, low-calorie diet; consistent physical activity; and complete avoidance of alcohol are also important, according to the NIH.

IS THIS A "CATCH-22" SITUATION?

Weight maintenance is beyond the scope of this book and readers are encouraged to explore the issues of holistic weight management through *Wings: Weight Success for a Lifetime* by Carol Simontacchi (see the reference section at the back of this book for contact information). Just know that following the "real food plan" presented in this book will go a long way toward solving weight issues without jeopardizing the health of the rest of the body. Weight management is not just a "mouth issue" or a "calories in/calories out" issue. The body has a very complex way of managing its calorie resources, and if we are going to solve our weight problem, we will have to approach weight management from a holistic perspective.

Abdominal Fat

You may have already heard about the "pear-shaped" woman, whose excess weight goes to her hips and thighs, and the "apple-shaped" woman, whose excess weight goes to her stomach and waist. Apple-shaped women face a greater risk of heart disease than their pear-shaped companions.

A report on the Nurses' Health Study confirmed that distribution of fat affects the risk for heart disease. Researchers included 44,702 women aged forty to sixty-five from 1986 to 1994 in the study. In 1986, these women had no history of heart disease, stroke, or cancer. They reported their waist and hip sizes to the researchers. After eight years, there were 320 documented cases of cardiovascular events (251 heart attacks and 69 deaths). Higher waist-to-hip ratios and bigger waist sizes were independently associated with a higher risk of coronary heart disease. Specifically, women with a waist-to-hip ratio of 0.88 or higher faced the greatest risk.

Being overweight and obese are significant issues for women of all ages, and the problem is growing each year. In our fast-paced culture that has no patience for home cooking and healthy meal choices, we are paying an extremely high price in uncontrolled weight. With added weight come added health challenges.

Most weight-loss programs on the market today tout a malnutrition-based diet, whether it is low calorie, low fat, high protein, or high carbohydrate.

As a result, dieters fail to lose weight, and each time they embark on another program, they become less likely to succeed (if success is measured by long-term maintenance of weight goals).

Weight-loss programs also contribute to hypothyroidism, female hormone imbalance, depression, insulin resistance (Syndrome X), and other health conditions that are precursors to heart disease. We really can say that dieting is a risk factor for heart disease—but so is obesity.

Diabetes

Women with Type 2 diabetes or insulin resistance face a three- to seven-fold risk for heart disease. In contrast, men with diabetes face a two- to three-fold increased risk. Some researchers speculate that the effect of diabetes on triglycerides and blood pressure is greater in women than in men.

African American, Hispanic, and Native American women with diabetes appear to face a greater risk of heart disease than women of other races. In fact, diabetes is one of the leading causes of death among the Native American population.

It should concern us, as a culture, to know that adult-onset diabetes is increasing in epidemic rates in children. As these children grow older, their risk of heart disease will skyrocket, as will other health concerns related to diabetes. Diabetes is the number five killer (heart disease is first, and cancer is second) in the U.S. As rates of diabetes rise, rates of heart disease will increase as well, since they are comorbid health conditions.

What causes Type 2 diabetes? According to standard medical philosophy, lack of physical activity, fatty diets, and excess weight are all associated with adult-onset diabetes. These three lifestyle/health factors certainly do play a role in the development of diabetes.

We cannot dismiss our love affair with sugar, however. The average American eats more than 200 pounds of sugar and artificial sweeteners per year, much of it in the form of soft drinks and candied cereals. But sugar isn't the only culprit. Highly processed carbohydrates that are high on the glycemic index are known to increase blood sugar disorders as well.

Consider the woman who eats a breakfast of a bowl of commercial granola, a piece of toast with a little jam or jelly, and a glass of orange juice; or a bagel with low-fat cream cheese; or a cup of coffee and a doughnut. Each one of these breakfast selections is comprised of little other than refined carbohydrates that cause spiraling blood sugar, a compensatory sudden release of insulin, and a following period of low blood sugar that drives the desire to eat more sugary foods. These types of meals directly contribute to the development of Syndrome X (to be discussed in a Chapter 3), and may boost the risk of diabetes as well.

We will discuss a healthy diet in Chapter 5. A moderate exercise program is also useful in reducing the risk of Type 2 diabetes.[18]

Other Risk Factors

- *African Americans.* Black women face a 69 percent higher risk of heart disease and stroke than white women. Factors may include socioeconomic status, access to medical care, genetics, and their particular physiology. Overall, African Americans have higher than average blood pressures, and a higher risk of fatal stroke, than whites. Prevention is critically important for African American women.[19]

- *Heredity.* If a close blood relative has had a heart attack or stroke, your risk increases.

- *Previous heart attacks or stroke.* If you've already had a heart attack or stroke, you face a higher risk of experiencing it again.

- *Periodontal disease.* Flossing may reduce heart attack risk for both women and men. Periodontal disease, also known as gum disease, occurs in more than half of American women and men. However, women appear to be more vulnerable to periodontal problems than men. Female hormones are to blame. When hormone levels are high—such as in menstruation, pregnancy, and menopause—the risk of periodontal problems increases, according to the American Dental Association.

  People with periodontal problems are believed to trigger small injuries that release bacteria into the bloodstream. They do this through normal activities such as brushing and chewing. The bacteria that cause periodontitis (inflammation of the gums) may generate blood clots and other proteins that can lead to heart attack and stroke.

PREVENTION PAYS

The following are guidelines for prevention of cardiovascular problems from the National Stroke Association and its panel of medical experts:

- Get your blood pressure checked at least once a year. If it's high, work with your doctor to lower it.
- Check for atrial fibrillation (irregular pulse). If you experience atrial fibrillation, work with your doctor to control it.
- If you smoke, quit.
- Drink alcohol in moderation or not at all.
- Get your cholesterol levels checked. If they're high (over 200 mg/dL overall), work with your doctor to lower them.
- If you have diabetes, work with your doctor to keep it under strict control.
- Get some physical activity most days of the week.
- Restrict your consumption of sodium and fat.
- Find out if you have circulation problems—another risk factor for stroke. If you do, work with your doctor to improve your circulation.

Rarely, periodontal bacteria can infect the lining or valves of the heart. This is known as infective endocarditis and usually happens in individuals who already have injured or abnormal valves.[20]

- *Medications.* Certain prescription or over-the-counter drugs may be contraindicated in women with heart disease. For example, Zoloft may pose a risk for women who've recently had a heart attack. The Food and Drug Administration (FDA) encourages anyone who knows of a serious adverse drug reaction to report it. You can visit www.fda.gov/medwatch and click on "How to Report," or you can call 1-800-FDA-1088.

Clearly, risk factors such as heredity, age, race, and gender cannot be controlled. Fortunately, there are many more factors that *can* be controlled, giving you greater mastery over your own health. (See Chapter 8 for more information.)

The Scourge of Ignorance

Perhaps the most prevalent risk factor for CVD and stroke is ignorance. Some women and men still postpone medical care because they don't recognize problematic symptoms, according to Harris Interactive, which conducted a national survey for the American Heart Association:

- Fewer than one in ten women surveyed considered heart disease their greatest health threat.
- Six of ten women surveyed identified cancer as their greatest health threat.
- Among women aged twenty-five to thirty-four, 72 percent believed that cancer is their greatest health threat, and only 4 percent recognized the danger of heart disease. Only 20 percent of this group understood that heart disease is the number-one killer of women.[21]
- In the year before the survey, only 20 percent of women surveyed had seen, heard, or read anything about heart disease in their doctors' offices. In addition, an estimated one-third of the 50 million people with high blood pressure in the U.S. do not realize they have it.[22]

Traditionally, it appears that doctors do not do enough to inform their female patients about heart disease symptoms and risks. The Harris Interactive survey, however, did find that 38 percent of women overall reported that their doctors started discussions on heart health. In 1997, that percentage was only 30 percent. Women who were forty-five to sixty-four years old witnessed the biggest change, from 38 percent in 1997 to 47 percent in 2000.

Informed female patients are more aware of their heart health and know what questions to ask their doctors.

What to Do

If you think you're having a heart attack, you or someone else must call 911 *immediately*. Every second counts. Delaying medical care could cost you your life.

In addition, take one aspirin, unless you have a sound medical reason for avoiding it. Aspirin is one of the safest, most affordable, and most helpful treatments immediately after a heart attack.

If you believe you are suffering from an ischemic stroke, you also need immediate medical care. Take a clot-busting medication such as t-PA as soon as possible. Do *not* take aspirin, however, which could worsen the condition.

It may also be helpful to cough. Oddly enough, coughing may stimulate the heart and help prevent further damage.

If all this information sounds scary, it shouldn't. It should sound *preventive*. Once we understand that women can suffer from cardiovascular disease, we can arm ourselves with the information to help prevent it. Just because we are vulnerable to a heart attack or stroke, it doesn't follow that we must succumb. We simply must be smarter; we must change our lives.

The information in the next chapters of this book will present very practical information about how to reduce our risk of heart disease. Just knowing the data, however, won't help. We'll have to make some serious efforts to change our diets and our lifestyles. We will need to work on our emotional and spiritual lives. But the process of taking charge of our health is a beneficial process. Part of healing is control, and we do have a great deal of control of most of the known risk factors for CVA. That is very good news, indeed.

CHAPTER 3

The Hormone Connection

OVER THE PAST FIFTY YEARS, technologists have developed an amazing worldwide communication system. We have desk telephones, wireless phones, fax machines, computers, navigational systems, and satellites. The complexity of the body's communication system makes our worldwide network look like a child's toy in comparison. Are you impressed with wireless communication? Our bodies were building wireless systems many millennia before someone discovered how to do it in your office. Your body has miles of "wires" that send messages at mind-blowing speeds. It's fabulous—when it works correctly.

When your body's communication system breaks down due to malfunction or malnutrition, however, chaos breaks loose.

Your body's communication system consists of the network of nerve tissues that receive and give messages from and to the brain and specific proteins manufactured in the endocrine and nervous systems. The nerves are the "wires," and there are miles of them in the human body. The body's wireless communication components are hormones and neurotransmitters, chemical bodies that float through the bloodstream and attach to receptor sites on cell walls, or burst across the synaptic gap between nerve cells.

The power of hormones cannot be underestimated. We women are familiar with our female hormonal systems "going haywire." We've experienced PMS, hot flashes, unstable moods, and chocolate cravings. We know about hormones!

The body produces many different hormones that communicate different messages. While these systems are separate and distinct, they work together. All the communication signals of the body must be working correctly (and in synchrony) if the entire body is to function normally. In the same way, if one hormone system malfunctions for any reason, all the systems are thrown into confusion, creating symptoms all over the body.

Neurotransmitters are equally important. These messengers are produced within nerve cells throughout the body, particularly the brain and the digestive system. Neurotransmitters relay signals between nerve cells at lightning speed and are kept in delicate balance by regulatory mechanisms within the nervous system itself. Hormones "talk" to the nervous system, and neurotransmitters communicate with the hormones. They all "talk" to each other.

All these communication systems "talk" to the cardiovascular and other body systems. Several hormones have a direct effect upon the health of the heart and arteries, so when we seek to improve heart health, we may want to start with the hormones. Cardiovascular health is, after all, a holistic issue.

How Female Hormones
Influence the Woman's Heart

We've known for a long time that female hormones (estrogen and progesterone) have a physiological effect on the heart.

Before the 1920s, physicians dispensed medicines made from animal glands. We still use these types of remedies, called glandulars. Glandulars contain tiny amounts of animal-derived hormones that are virtually identical to human hormones and serve a physiological purpose.

In the 1920s, scientists discovered how to isolate estrogen and progesterone in the laboratory. Use of estrogen replacement therapy (ERT) was limited throughout the 1930s and 1940s, but from the 1950s until 2001, American physicians routinely prescribed ERT or hormone replacement therapy (HRT) for menopausal women. Menopause was considered an estrogen-deficiency disease, and supplemental estrogen seemed like the obvious solution. Besides addressing menopausal symptoms (hot flashes, night sweats, mood swings, vaginal dryness), HRT was thought to protect against heart disease and bone loss. In addition, women were told that estrogen would make them look more youthful and attractive.[1]

Although the benefits of estrogen seemed clear, its risks were poorly understood. In 1975, the first negative reports about estrogen therapy emerged. The medical literature began to show a link between estrogen use and endometrial cancer (cancer of the lining of the uterus). The research indicated that women who used estrogen therapy were four and a half times more susceptible to this type of cancer.[2]

The Progestin Factor

Subsequent research showed that adding progestins to the estrogen proto-col reduced cancer risk. Progestins are synthetic forms of the human hormone progesterone. In a 1978 study, 139 perimenopausal and postmen-opausal women were treated for endometrial hyperplasia (precancerous lesions of the lining of the uterus). When treated with progestins, the hyper-plasia reverted back to healthy tissue in 133 patients.[3]

In the mid-1970s, the medical community discovered that postmenopausal women who took estrogen were four to ten times more likely to develop endometrial cancer. To combat the effects of estrogen, they added progestin, shown to significantly reduce the risk of this cancer.[4]

Estrogen therapy became estrogen-progestin therapy, or hormone replace-ment therapy (HRT). In the 1980s and most of the 1990s, large studies sup-ported the benefits of pharmaceutical HRT. These studies indicated that women on HRT had fewer heart attacks and strokes than women who weren't on it.

Even then, however, some skeptics cited weaknesses in the research. Other factors may have been responsible for the apparent benefits of HRT. For example, data suggests that women on HRT are, in general, more health conscious. They are less likely to smoke, more likely to be well educated, and more likely to exercise consistently and eat a balanced diet.[5] Each of these lifestyle factors reduces the risk of heart disease.

For decades, women were routinely offered HRT, even when they were relatively free from menopausal symptoms, as a supposed preventive meas-ure against the development of heart disease and osteoporosis. But when newer research began raising the specter of serious side effects such as can-cer, the medical community and women were thrown into confusion. Should women be placed on HRT or shouldn't they? Is it safe, or does it increase the risk of death from other causes?

Researchers, physicians, and women are finding that there is, indeed, a dark side to ERT or HRT. It does not confer protection against heart disease, either.

The Dramatic About-Face

In 2001, the American Heart Association (AHA) advised doctors to stop pre-scribing hormone replacement therapy (HRT) to women to prevent heart disease. Further, the AHA stated that healthy women should not be told that taking estrogen may protect the heart.[6]

In addition, the AHA advised doctors to stop estrogen treatment immediately in postmenopausal women who have had heart attacks. (Women who have a history of heart disease, and who are on HRT, should speak with their doctors about the pros and cons of continuing HRT). The advisory was published as a result of several studies indicating that women on HRT have the same risk of heart attack as women not on it. Doctors have been prescribing HRT under the false assumption that it would protect women's hearts. Since HRT's efficacy for heart health is highly questionable, women need to find other routes to heart health, which we will explore in this book.

The Heart and Estrogen-Progestin Replacement Study (HERS) burst the bubble. HERS was a double-blind, placebo-controlled, randomized trial on estrogen-progestin treatment and women with coronary artery disease (CAD). The study was conducted in seventeen clinics across the country, with 2,763 patients. The women either took estrogen derived from horse urine (Premarin) alone or estrogen with a progestin. For more than four years, the project staff closely monitored the cardiovascular and gynecological health of the study participants.

The results raised some eyebrows. After four-plus years, no significant differences in cardiovascular events were found between the control group and the placebo group. Two distinct time trends were identified, however. In the first year, the HRT group experienced more cardiovascular events than the control group. As time passed, however, the placebo group faced a higher rate of these adverse events.[7]

In some studies, HRT appears to have no effect on artery blockage. In one trial, researchers performed angiographies to assess arterial blockage in more than three hundred individuals with CAD. The women in the study were randomly given 0.625 mg of conjugated estrogen daily; 0.625 mg of conjugated estrogen, plus 2.5 mg of medroxyprogesterone acetate daily; or a placebo daily. Two assessments were done: one at the beginning of the study and one at the end, more than three years later.

Both groups significantly lowered their LDL cholesterol levels (the "harmful" cholesterol), and increased their HDL (beneficial) levels. However, neither treatment changed the progression of coronary atherosclerosis. The number of cardiovascular events was similar in both groups. The researchers concluded that women with established heart disease should not expect a cardiovascular benefit from HRT.[8]

HRT does not appear to protect against stroke, either. In another trial, the 2,763 postmenopausal women from HERS were randomly assigned to take conjugated estrogen plus progestin or a placebo. After four years, 149 women had one or more strokes, resulting in 26 deaths. HRT did not appear to affect the risk of stroke in postmenopausal women with coronary artery disease.[9]

Researchers were surprised by the results of HERS. They had started the trial with the expectation that hormone replacement therapy would protect heart health, and ended it with a completely different result.[10]

Another study, even more frightening, suggested that women who started HRT after experiencing a heart attack were 44 percent more likely than women who had never tried HRT to have another heart attack or die in the following year. The study involved nearly 1,900 postmenopausal women who had experienced heart attacks.[11]

Aborted Study

The National Heart, Lung, and Blood Institute (NHLBI), along with other sectors of the National Institutes of Health (NIH), began the Women's Health Initiative (WHI) Study in 1991. It involved more than 161,000 healthy, postmenopausal women. One of its purposes was to evaluate the long-term impact of HRT on heart disease, osteoporosis, and breast cancer.

THE GENE QUESTION

Dr. Bruce M. Psaty of the University of Washington in Seattle asks a significant question about the recent studies on HRT and heart disease. He speculates that certain women may have a genetic mutation that puts them at higher risk of heart disease. He and his colleagues investigated the impact of mutations in the genes for factor V and prothrombin, two blood-clotting factors.

The study involved 232 postmenopausal women who had already experienced a heart attack, and 723 postmenopausal women who had not. The women were checked for mutations in the genes for the two blood-clotting factors.

The researchers speculate that the gene mutation may interact with HRT to increase heart attack risk. However, only eight women in the study were on HRT, had high blood pressure, and had the prothrombin gene mutation. Clearly, more research is required.[12, 13]

This part of the study was expected to continue until 2005. In 2002, however, the WHI Data and Safety Monitoring Board (DSMB) recommended that study participants taking estrogen and progestin stop taking their pills. After noting an increased risk for heart attack, strokes, blood clots, and breast cancer in these women, the researchers concluded that the risks overshadowed the benefits. The WHI continues to study women who take estrogen only at this time, though.

The controversy rages on and will probably persist as science continues to present conflicting results. The only question that is germane to you the reader is, "What is best for me?" That question may be difficult to answer. The most we may be able to do is present the information and let you make the decision with your personal physician.

What About Progesterone?

Estrogen isn't the only female hormone—it isn't even the most vital one. In the context of the discussion of heart health and female hormones, it will be instructive to look at the role of estrogen's sister hormone, progesterone. What may be most important to this discussion is not so much whether estrogen or progesterone are beneficial, but whether estrogen and progesterone are kept within a normal physiological balance. It is important for each hormone to function within the parameters set by a healthy body, and that this balance remain steady throughout the perimenopausal and menopausal periods of life.

What is progesterone? How do estrogen and progesterone work together? How do they work in opposition to each other?

Sister Hormones

Estrogen is released by the ovaries, although some estrogen is produced in the adrenal glands and by body fat. It remains the dominant female hormone for the first fourteen days of the menstrual cycle. (The start of menstrual flow is day one of the menstrual cycle.) Estrogen begins to rise at the beginning of the cycle, reaching a climax around day seven. At this point, the concentration of estrogen in the tissue begins to diminish.

Progesterone is the dominant hormone during the second half of the menstrual cycle, and aids in gestation, should pregnancy occur. Progesterone begins to rise about day fifteen of the cycle, reaching a climax around day twenty-one. Then it begins to recede as the cycle reaches its conclusion and prepares for another cycle around day twenty-eight. The corpus luteum, the tiny vesicle that produces and drops an egg each month, manufactures progesterone. When the egg is released into the fallopian tubes, the corpus luteum releases progesterone that helps sustain the pregnancy if the egg meets a sperm on its way down the fallopian tube.

Often, during puberty, after childbirth, or in perimenopause, these normal estrogen/progesterone cycles are thrown into chaos, leading to physical and mental/emotional symptoms and an increased risk of heart disease.

THE POWER OF ESTROGEN

Estrogen is actually a family of hormones. Perhaps two dozen different forms of the hormone, each with a different molecular structure, may be produced and used by the body, each serving a different function. Estrogen receptors can be found in the brain, heart, liver, and on virtually every part of the human body. Men produce estrogen as well, but in far lower amounts than do women.

How powerful is estrogen? The average woman produces about one tablespoon of the hormone in her entire lifetime. Estrogen is physiologically active in parts per billion (nanogram amounts).

Interestingly, although estriol has displayed the potential to prevent cancer, it is not used in the United States in hormone replacement therapy. And although phytoestrogens (plant-derived estrogens) have been shown to be effective, they are largely ignored in this country. Why?

The answer is simple—and sad. Bioidentical plant hormones cannot be patented, and therefore are not considered profitable. The pharmaceutical industry, unfortunately, is devoted to profit, not to public health.[14]

The most abundant forms of estrogen are estrone, estradiol, and estriol. (In contrast, Premarin is composed of 48 percent estrones and 52 percent horse estrogens.) Estrones are converted in the body to estradiol—the form of estrogen most strongly associated with increased cancer risk.

When a woman becomes anovulatory (no longer producing an egg each month), her body may no longer manufacture enough progesterone to balance out the estrogen. Furthermore, women are exposed to environmental estrogens, called *xenoestrogens*, that unbalance the two natural hormones. This leads to a relative dominance of estrogen in relation to progesterone. Nutrient deficiencies or excesses can also disrupt the normal estrogen/progesterone balance, particularly during the postpartum period, or in women who have dieted frequently.

According to John Lee, M.D., author and retired physician, it is the imbalance between estrogen and progesterone that causes all the trouble. Some symptoms typical of dominant estrogen include acceleration of the aging process, depression, increased blood clotting, fat gain (especially around the abdomen, hips, and thighs), and thyroid dysfunction mimicking hypothyroidism.[15] Each of these symptoms is a risk factor for the development of cardiovascular disease. For more information about the female hormone connection to heart disease, you may wish to read Dr. Lee's excellent book, *What Your Doctor May Not Tell You About Menopause.* (Warner Books, 1996).

Estrogen dominance is also linked to insulin resistance and obesity, two more markers for heart disease.

According to Dr. Lee, progesterones and progestins are not synonymous. They are not structurally identical and do not have the same effects on the body. In a nutshell, Dr. Lee claims that adding progestin (instead of progesterone) to a hormone pill does not help to restore the natural estrogen/progesterone balance. He notes that some of the effects of combined estrogen and progestin therapy may include increased blood pressure, headaches, changes in sex drive, and hypothyroidism.

Naturally occurring progesterone is heart protective and reduces other risk factors for heart disease as well, such as obesity and hypothyroidism. Clinicians have found that when natural estrogen and natural progesterone are combined in a balanced and cyclical pattern that mimics nature's own hormone balance, the heart and arteries are protected, lowering the risk of heart disease.

If Not HRT, Then What?

Certainly, natural hormone balance is integral to heart health. It increases HDL cholesterol while lowering LDL cholesterol. It lowers blood pressure, and enhances the health of the thyroid gland. It helps reduce obesity and obesity-related illnesses. It decreases insulin resistance, one of the most important risk factors for the development of heart disease. That's why a woman's risk of heart disease before menopause—when her body is still producing sufficient estrogen—is lower than a man's. Even though a woman's risk increases after menopause, at least 40 percent of her longer life expectancy can be traced back to her early protection against heart disease.[16]

Today, American physicians are less likely to recommend HRT to their postmenopausal patients who have heart disease. Instead, they are beginning to emphasize other protective measures: quitting smoking; controlling blood pressure, cholesterol, and blood sugar; and sticking with a consistent exercise program.

Despite the risks associated with pharmaceutical HRT, death from heart disease has fallen 60 to 70 percent over the last thirty-plus years. This decrease is, indeed, heartening. Heart disease is still the leading cause of death across the United States, however, claiming nearly three-quarters of a million lives per year.[17] Author and physician Christine Northrup, M.D., points out, "Cardiovascular disease is epidemic in this culture in part because of lifestyle and diet, not estrogen deficiency disease."[18] The decreased rate of heart disease coincides with growing awareness of preventive health measures, a fact that is not surprising.

The Little Giant

While we are talking about hormones that affect female physiology, especially the heart, we must include a discussion about the critically important thyroid hormone. We call the thyroid gland the "little giant" because it wields such a huge influence over the human body. The most active form of thyroid hormone is T3; T4 converts into T3 in a healthy body and helps maintain healthy levels of the active hormone.

The influence of thyroid hormone on the body and other organs is incredibly widespread. When the thyroid gland is removed from an otherwise normal animal, all metabolic activity is reduced. In humans, the metabolic rate can be reduced up to 40 percent, and at this rate, excess amounts of water, salt, and protein are retained in the body. Blood cholesterol increases as well.

The symptoms of hypothyroidism can include fatigue, an abnormal apron of fat, weakness, inability to lose weight, lethargy, edema (water retention), decreased sweating, thick tongue, thinning hair, coarseness of the hair, constipation, depression, intolerance to temperature changes, goiter, hoarse speech, dry skin, coarse skin, slow speech, sensation of cold, cold skin, pallor of the skin, impaired memory, elevated cholesterol, and anxiety.

Hypothyroidism causes mental and emotional problems such as poor memory, nervousness, irritability, impaired abstract thinking and psychological performance, problems with attention, and slow intellectual performance.

The thyroid appears to act in concert with estrogen. Thyroid hormone helps break down excessive estrogens, and often female complaints can be resolved easily by handling the thyroid problem. Women who simultaneously use estrogen replacement therapy and thyroid replacement therapy may not be getting the benefits of the thyroid therapy, because increased estrogen lowers thyroid levels in women. According to an article in the *New England Journal of Medicine*, "increases in estrogen such as those that occur in pregnancy, lead to dips in thyroid levels. Among women with normal thyroid function, the gland can compensate and produce more thyroid hormone. But this barometer does not work in women with hypothyroidism. The author recommends that women receiving both types of hormone replacement have their thyroid levels checked within twelve weeks of starting on estrogen—particularly women who are on thyroid hormone as part of thyroid cancer treatment."[19]

Thyroid hormone affects blood sugar levels, too. The thyroid controls the utilization of glucose within the cells, and maintains feedback control over the other hormones involved in glucose conversion in the cells, muscles, and liver. When thyroid hormone is low, the production of hormones (such as glucagon from the pancreas and adrenal hormones, including cortisone, glucocorticosteroids, and mineralcorticoids) is slowed and cannot function as well. The resulting symptoms include increased water retention, reduced ability to burn stored sugars (triglycerides) as energy, and increased production of damaging ketone bodies.

Interestingly, virtually every diet on the market today affects the thyroid, and not to its benefit. Low-fat diets slow metabolism, as do high-protein and high-carbohydrate diets. Low-calorie diets make the body feel as though famine were reducing the food supply, and the thyroid slows the metabolism of the body to conserve energy.

Certain environmental toxins harm the thyroid, such as organophosphates, carbamates, OCCs, fungicides, PCBs, and mercury. Diets that contain large amounts of soy may cause goiter, or slowed thyroid function. It would appear that everywhere we turn, some environmental, dietary, or biochemical stimuli is working against our thyroid glands, which in turn affects all the other organs of the endocrine system.

How does hypothyroidism affect the heart? It increases water retention, cholesterol, and triglycerides, adds fat deposition (overweight), and unbalances the female hormones, thereby adding to the risk of cardiovascular disease. It also increases blood sugar disorders, which can heighten the occurrence of insulin resistance.

The Role of Insulin and Other Hormones

Estrogen, progesterone, and the thyroid hormone are not the only hormones involved in cardiovascular health. Another biochemical messenger is the hormone insulin, produced in the pancreas. Insulin is released when blood sugar levels are too high, pulling the excess sugars into the liver for short-term storage, or into fat tissue for long-term storage. If the pancreas does not manufacture any—or enough—insulin, diabetes develops.

People with diabetes face an increased risk of coronary artery disease. Robert H. Eckel, M.D., professor of medicine at the University of Colorado Health Science Center, states, "Atherosclerotic damage to the coronary arteries is two to four times more common in asymptomatic people with Type 1 diabetes than in the general population."[20]

The standard American diet (SAD) promotes blood glucose imbalances and Type 2 (adult-onset) diabetes. The average American now consumes an average of 152 pounds of sugar per year, in addition to many more pounds of synthetic sweeteners. These levels are too high for the body to manage. American women on a carbohydrate binge typically fill up on sweets or other refined carbohydrates, and those processed sugars barge into the bloodstream. The pancreas overreacts by pumping excess insulin into the bloodstream, reducing glucose levels and leading to symptoms of low blood sugar (light-headedness, irritability, and confusion).

When that happens, the adrenal glands get involved. In response to low blood sugar levels, the adrenals flood the system with another hormone—adrenaline—to pull glucose levels back up. In the short term, the adrenal glands can do this without any difficulty. Over the long term, however, they can become exhausted. The blood sugar control mechanisms are then thrown out of balance.

Syndrome X

One of the most common markers for heart disease is a condition called *Syndrome X* (also known as metabolic syndrome or insulin resistance). One theory asserts that Syndrome X is genetically based. Women and men most at risk for Syndrome X have excessive fat around the abdomen, high triglycerides, low HDL cholesterol, and high blood pressure, according to the American Heart Association.

How does insulin resistance develop, and why is it becoming more widespread? Obesity appears to be the primary culprit. More than 80 percent of people with Type 2 diabetes are obese. It is no accident that while the rate of obesity in this country is increasing, so is the rate of Type 2 diabetes. It used to be called "adult-onset" diabetes, but more young people are developing it because of the dramatic rise of childhood obesity over the past two decades.[21]

In individuals with Type 2 diabetes, or in other carbohydrate-sensitive, nondiabetic people, the body's cells gradually become more resistant to insulin. In a healthy person, when insulin binds to a cell, it sends a message to glucose transporters to push glucose into the cell and out of the bloodstream. However, when people become resistant to insulin, that message is blocked, and the cells are unable to take in sufficient glucose from the blood. As a result, blood sugar levels rise, and the pancreas is forced to manufacture yet more insulin. More and more insulin floods the bloodstream, damaging the delicate cardiovascular system and increasing the risk of heart disease. The insulin resistance gradually grows stronger as the pancreas grows weaker. Finally, blood sugar levels rise and lead to symptoms of Type 2 diabetes. In true Syndrome X, diabetes doesn't necessarily develop—but an increased risk of heart disease does.

Symptoms of insulin resistance and Type 2 diabetes include the following:

1. Greater thirst and urination
2. Less energy and more appetite
3. Weight loss
4. Eye damage
5. Pain and tingling sensations
6. Loss of consciousness and disorientation

The relatively recent discovery of a hormone called resistin sheds new light on insulin resistance. Resistin seems to promote insulin resistance, and researchers speculate that it may be the direct link between obesity and Type 2 diabetes.[22]

It appears that obesity generates higher levels of resistin in the body. In one editorial, the author points out that administration of an antiresistin antibody improved blood sugar and insulin action in obese mice.[23]

Damage to the Heart

How does Syndrome X, or insulin resistance, damage the cardiovascular system? Out-of-control blood sugar leads to a buildup of fatty substances in the blood vessels. The thicker these blood vessels become, the less blood they supply. The accumulation of plaque in the blood vessel results in atherosclerosis.

Because the body's cells are getting less blood and oxygen, people with insulin resistance face a higher risk of damage to the heart, brain, legs, kidneys, nerves, and skin. Poor circulation also impairs wound healing, increasing the risk of stroke, gangrene of the hands and feet, erectile dysfunction, and infections.

How widespread is the problem of Syndrome X? It is very common, according to researcher Gerald Reaven, M.D., author of *Syndrome X, the Silent Killer* (Fireside, 2001) is increasing in epidemic proportions in the American population because of our love affair with sugar, soft drinks, processed fats, and other high glycemic foods (potatoes, white rice, corn, and so on).

Take a look at the general shape of the population, particularly women, and you'll see just how common Syndrome X is. Individuals who are insulin resistant tend to hang onto excess weight around the stomach and abdomen, producing protruded bellies that mimic the look of pregnancy. They carry excess weight around the upper body as well, one of the markers for heart disease.

Syndrome X is not a benign disorder. It is a serious risk factor for heart disease, and women are just as susceptible as men.

Leptin

Another hormone, leptin, is drawing increased interest from researchers. Leptin, the hormonal link between adipose (fat) tissue and the nervous system, is produced in the body's fat cells. Leptin helps regulate obesity. Earlier studies found that mice that were missing the gene that regulates leptin production became fat. Paradoxically, researchers have found high leptin levels in obese individuals. They speculate that these individuals are leptin resistant, rendering their systems incapable of responding to the hormone.

The role of leptin in obesity is controversial. Some research indicates that certain obese individuals have a genetic mutation that leads to low levels of leptin. In some cases, injections of leptin have resulted in a normalized appetite and weight loss.

However, researcher Stephen O'Rahilly, M.D., speculates, "It has been clear that most obese people do not have an absolute deficiency in leptin,"[25] and "The findings suggest that moderate reductions in plasma leptin might actually have an influence on fat mass, tending to push it up."[26]

METABOLISM AND INSULIN RESISTANCE

At least one review suggests that waning thermogenic function (metabolism) contributes to obesity-related hypertension. The author speculates that as subjects age, it becomes more difficult to metabolize foods. Obesity and insulin resistance may result. Of course, obesity is a primary risk factor for hypertension and other cardiovascular ailments.

The author cautions, however, "Hypertension is rarely the consequence of a single mechanism."[24]

Research has also shown that, surprisingly, blood levels of leptin are higher in hypertensive individuals of normal weight than in people who have normal weight and normal blood pressure.[27]

One study examined 263 women and 133 men under the age of sixty-five, who did not have diabetes and who were not taking medications for high blood pressure. Researchers adjusted for age, body mass index, and insulin. They found higher diastolic blood pressure (the pressure when the heart is resting between beats) among men with higher leptin levels. Furthermore, researchers found significantly higher plasma leptin levels in insulin-resistant women than in insulin-sensitive men, regardless of hypertension.[28] Obviously, more research is necessary before making a definitive recommendation.

What Are We Going to Do About It?

First, let's deal with the question of female hormones. Fortunately, most women do not require prescription medications to get through menopause. Nourishing the female system may, however, require extra diligence because of the stressful lives we all lead. We will read in Chapter 4 that stress is extremely damaging to the cardiovascular system because of excessive secretions of the stress hormone cortisol. Cortisol causes elevated blood pressure and other cardiovascular symptoms. When estrogen levels are high, stress hormone levels soar, up to two to three times the normal range, paving another pathway to estrogen-related heart conditions. Stress unbalances the female hormone system.

In addition, we are bathed in xenoestrogens (synthetic estrogens from the environment). Because xenoestrogens are everywhere, it is nearly impossible to avoid the physiological effects of these synthetics.

We've been saturated with information about plant-based estrogens called phytoestrogens, found in soy foods, red clover, and other food products. The nutriceutical industry spikes many processed foods with phytoestogens, such as daidzen and genestein, in an attempt to raise estrogen levels. This decision is based on the mistaken belief that estrogen deficiency is causing the trouble. The problem with soy-based foods is that they can create their own unique biochemical imbalances, such as hypothyroidism, decreased mineral absorption, and allergy problems. The problem of hormone imbalance is more complicated than just popping a soy pill or adding a cup of soymilk to your breakfast cereal.

Restoring Hormone Balance

So, what are we going to do to "fix" our inner telecommunications system? While the system is complicated, it may not be so difficult to restore hormonal balance. Frankly, that is what the body wants to do. Restoring homeostasis (balance) is well within the body's natural ability, *if* we give the body the proper tools with which to work.

To restore homeostasis, we must get our minds out of the drug mentality mode. As we mentioned, menopause is not a disease and does not usually require medication. Syndrome X, while serious, is relatively simple to correct with diet, exercise, and supplementation alone.

Certainly, the studies can be confusing, and we wonder if we will ever be able to get our arms around this problem and tackle it. However, all we need to do is feed the body. The body will usually do the rest.

Herbs can be helpful in balancing female hormones, such as chaste tree berry (vitex), dong quai, black cohosh, and others. Purchase an herb book and study the natural pharmacy that was designed to restore homeostasis to the female body. (See the reference section in the back of this book for a list of recommended herb reference books.) If possible, consult a nutritionally trained physician who can provide further information about balancing hormones.

If hormone replacement therapy is needed for severe menopausal symptons, speak to your physician about using natural hormones that mimic the body's own twenty-eight-day cycle, with forms of the hormones that mimic the body's own. Many physicians collaborate with a compounding pharmacist who can construct an estrogen and progesterone prescription to work with your body. Other physicians recommend the use of a progesterone cream for two weeks out of every month, to mimic the body's own hormonal cycle. (Again, Dr. Lee's book provides valuable information about how to balance hormones effectively.)

Treating hypothyroidism is not a do-it-yourself project. Many clinicians believe that even diagnosing hypothyroidism can be tricky, especially if one is relying solely on blood tests of T3 and T4 values. Many clinicians recommend a three-pronged approach to an accurate diagnosis of thyroid problems. (Remember that low progesterone levels mask low T3 levels. When progesterone levels are low, you may experience the symptoms of hypothyroidism. However, the T3 and T4 levels in the blood will remain normal, leading to a possible misdiagnosis of hypothyroidism. Check with your doctor.) Body temperature is a useful barometer of metabolism, especially when the basal temperature is taken several times during the day, over a period of several days. Normal temperature should be 98.6 degrees; a lowered temperature of more than half of a degree may signal low thyroid.

Check the list of thyroid-deficiency symptoms to see how many pertain to you. Take the list of deficiency symptoms, along with a chart of body temperature, to your physician and ask him for a blood panel that includes several measures of thyroid function. Putting this information together may be a more accurate way of measuring thyroid function than simply measuring the amount of thyroid hormone in the blood.

Nourishing the thyroid gland is very important. Remember that the thyroid hormone is synthesized from the amino acid tyrosine. Make sure your diet is adequate in this essential amino acid (vegetarians may have low levels of tyrosine), along with vitamin B_6 and trace amounts of iodine. Before going on thyroid hormone, ask your physician if using 100 mg of tyrosine, along with vitamin B_6, may assist in the manufacture of thyroid hormone, thereby boosting thyroid hormone levels naturally.

Reduce the consumption of goitrogens such as soy and foods in the brassica family (cabbage, kale, and others).

Reducing Syndrome X

Reducing the risk of developing Syndrome X, or reversing Syndrome X, is not difficult, provided you are willing to make significant dietary and lifestyle changes. Review the information in Chapter 5 about a healthy diet, and begin eating like a cavewoman. In other words, consume lots of vegetables, lots of fiber, and lots of water. Ingest small amounts of fresh fruit. Get good sources of protein balanced in three regular meals per day. Choose raw, natural fats such as olive oil, raw nuts and seeds, and avocados.

You already know the list of dietary no-no's that caused the problem in the first place: sugar, soft drinks, processed fats (hydrogenated fats such as margarine), and foods high on the glycemic index list (potatoes, white rice, corn, bread, pasta, cereal, and other grain foods). Ease them out of the diet.

Keep in mind that the typical American breakfast—a cup of coffee and a bagel with low-fat cream cheese—only hastens the development of Syndrome X. So does a bowl of sugary cereal moistened with milk and a piece of toast. Even worse? A cup of coffee, glass of orange juice, and a donut. *Mainly, we simply must reduce the sugars in our diets!*

One of the best ways to balance blood sugar in the morning is to enjoy a breakfast drink of 100 percent rice protein powder, 1 tablespoon of olive oil, and fresh fruit such as bananas or strawberries, blended with water. A complete breakfast in a glass can help reduce blood sugar and decrease insulin resistance.

Making up for years of bad eating habits and reversing insulin resistance will require supplementation. Review the supplement recommendations in Chapter 6. Make sure you are getting enough chromium (used to activate insulin), magnesium (needed to metabolize sugar and normalize blood sugar levels), zinc (used to metabolize sugar and normalize blood sugar), and vanadium (mimics the action of insulin).

CHAPTER 4

The Broken Heart of a Woman

ARE WOMEN TRULY FRAGILE? We have been called the weaker sex, but that's not really true. Female bodies may not be as strong as male bodies (our lower testosterone levels diminish muscle mass). But it sure seems like we handle a lot of stress and a lot of grief, and we just keep on taking care of the family. Our hearts just go on pumping.

Poets and lovers know about broken hearts, and doctors know that broken hearts can fail. In other words, we *can* die of a broken heart. Stress and depression can cut our lives short, in a very real sense.

More and more women struggle with day-to-day stress and depression, which are gradually killing them. In fact, studies show that depression and stress are increasing at exponential rates. If the current trend continues, these factors will become the number-one killer around the world, even in our affluent society.

When Does Life Get Easier?

Long ago, in another era, wives played just one role: homemaker. Yes, that title conferred a lot of work, including caring for the children, husband, and house. It was also a very confining, restrictive role that must have driven some women nearly crazy.

Several decades ago, as technology took a more prominent role in the home, inventors promised women an easier life. All they had to do was to accumulate lots of work-saving gadgets.

Well, now women have automatic washing machines, electric or gas ranges, food processors, vacuum cleaners, and indoor plumbing. How easy can life get?

But if our houses are crammed with so many time-saving, work-saving gadgets, why are we working even harder than our mothers? I remember my mother relaxing as she stitched embroidery designs on her pillowcases and replaced missing buttons on her man's trousers. She was working, but she was relaxing, too.

Maybe we work hard so we can pay for all that stuff. It doesn't make sense, does it?

Stress is not the only emotional pressure on our hearts, however. As a nation of women, we are sad. Depression is overwhelming us, in increasingly higher numbers and in increasing severity.

STRESS SYMPTOMS

Psychological symptoms of stress include tension, anger, anxiety, reclusiveness, feelings of pessimism or cynicism, irritability or resentfulness, and an inability to focus or perform at the normal level. Physical symptoms include frequent headaches, fatigue, insomnia, digestive upset, skin problems, neck or back pain, loss of appetite, overeating, or excessive drinking.[1]

Depression is often called the "common cold" of the mental health world. Women suffer from mental disorders, particularly depression, in far higher numbers than men. One explanation may be that men are less likely to report symptoms of depression and seek treatment for it.

Some of women's mental suffering may be due to hormonal imbalances. Overwork and underplay are a big part of depression, too. We women work too hard and don't laugh enough. Depression is a significant risk factor in the onset and progression of cardiovascular disease.

Rising Abuse of Children and Women

Perhaps one of the reasons for our crushing depression and stress is a history of sexual, emotional, and/or physical abuse. Our hearts are breaking as we carry around a burden of unresolved abuse that can span decades. We store our grief in our hearts. Studies show that abuse is not a small problem; it is a very large problem, and not in just the lower echelons of society. Abuse strikes upper-class, middle-class, and lower-class families in just about the same percentages. The statistics are hideous.

It's possible that more than half of our society may have suffered or may be suffering from some type of severe abuse within a family relationship, suggests Vincent Felitti, M.D. of the Southern California Permanente Medical

Group in San Diego, California. In a study performed in San Diego (a middle-to upper-class community) on more than 13,000 adults who completed a standardized medical evaluation at a large HMO, more than 70 percent responded. Out of these 70 percent, more than half reported at least one exposure to abuse, and one-fourth reported more than two exposures to childhood abuse. Dr. Felitti noted a strong relationship to the presence of adult diseases in these abuse survivors, including a higher risk of ischemic heart disease.[2]

Abuse frequently begins early in childhood, and the effects of the assault continue into adulthood. Unless true healing takes place, recovery from the original injury never happens. The victims never truly heal. Studies show that adults who were abused as children are more vulnerable to excessive moodiness, irritability, depression, or angry outbursts. They may be emotionally numb and unable to respond to affection, and may experience disturbing flashbacks. Survivors of childhood abuse may be incapable of appreciating the present.[3]

We seldom, however, associate these "difficult personalities" with difficulties in childhood. We seldom attribute our personal irritability, depression, angry outbursts, or moodiness to emotional and/or physical injuries inflicted in our youth. Few of us seek professional help for moodiness; we just try to control our temperament. We "stuff" our feelings—but the feelings do not go away. They eat away at our hearts and bodies. We succumb to heart disease because our hearts were broken when we were young.

We know that childhood abuse causes permanent changes to the brain, including:

- Increased incidence of epileptic seizures, caused by changes to the limbic system (the part of the brain that controls emotions).
- Increased incidence of abnormal EEG, associated with increased self-destructive behavior and aggression.
- Deficient development of the left side of the brain, leading to depression and problems with memory. Moreover, integration problems occur between the left and right sides of the brain, because of a decrease in the size of the bridge between the two hemispheres.

Additionally, abuse creates changes in hormones and neurotransmitters. According to one researcher, "We know that an animal exposed to stress and neglect early in life develops a brain that is wired to experience fear, anxiety, and stress. We think the same is true of people."[4]

Are women targeted for abuse? It often appears so. Women are more susceptible than men to sexual harassment, sexual abuse, and physical abuse.[5] Research indicates that three out of five depressed women have been victims of sexual and/or physical abuse.[6] In one case-control study, 732 women, ages 36 to 45, completed a self-administered questionnaire that focused on their history of violent victimization. Half (363) of the women experienced or feared abuse as a child or adolescent. Sixty-eight of the 732 women reported violence as an adult only. Not surprisingly, the highest rates of depression were found in women who were severely victimized in childhood or adolescence.[7]

Psychopathology is not the only health consequence of past or continual abuse. Physiological changes occur as well, as increased cortisol (stress hormone) floods the system, damaging the heart and the brain. Exaggerated cortisol responses increase blood pressure, speed the heart rate, unbalance blood sugar, and increase the risk of Syndrome X and diabetes (among the most dramatic precursors to heart disease).

Research clearly indicates that childhood abuse increases the risk of numerous disease states, including certain forms of heart disease. Childhood abuse also increases the risk of psychological disease.

INHERITED DEPRESSION

Certain types of depression may be inherited. If you have a first-degree relative (parents, siblings) who suffers from depression, you have a 25 percent risk of developing it.[8]

Past emotional/physical/sexual abuse is a killer—particularly a killer of women.

Is Marriage Protective—or Harmful?

Remember the saying, "Better to have loved and lost than never to have loved at all"? That sweet sentiment doesn't hold up to scientific scrutiny. It may be far healthier to remain single than to suffer through a bad marriage.

Psychologist and author John Gottman, Ph.D., states:

> When people love and they make a commitment, they become enormously vulnerable and enormously powerful—because they care so much

and it connects them to the world in such a big way. That is the amazing thing about all these benefits: They are conferred by commitment. The commitment is like falling over backward and translates into making you a mensch and a secure human being—somebody who is involved in the community of mankind.[9]

A miserable marriage, however, is another story. A bad marriage is a key contributing factor to both anxiety and depression. It appears that an unhappy union breaks a heart in more ways than one. Marital problems can speed the heart rate, increase blood pressure, and trigger a flood of cortisol.

The stress of a bad marriage is even more acute in women who already have heart disease. Living in a hurtful environment makes heart disease even worse, increasing the risk of having a heart attack or developing unstable angina pectoris more than twofold. Even when live-in couples are unmarried, an unhappy union will more than double the women's risk of a heart event, compared to women living alone.[10]

Are Single People Healthier?

What about single people? The Minnesota Heart Survey yielded some interesting results. The survey involved more than 7,800 midwestern men and women. The authors of the survey found that separated or divorced people had the highest rate of hospitalization for a heart attack or stroke. Married people showed a low rate for hospitalization; widowed people reported an intermediate rate. The hospitalization rate for never-married people was as low or lower than that of married people.[11]

According to a report from the World Health Organization (WHO), however, marriage appears to be more protective for men than for women. Higher rates of depression were found in married women. Husbands aren't necessarily to blame. Women who choose to work inside the home often face a monotonous routine, loneliness, little intellectual stimulation, and lack of personal income. Furthermore, the role of the housewife is not as respected as it once was. This factor alone may deplete a woman's self-esteem.[12] The isolation of the twenty-first-century housewife is unique to this culture and this time.

Stay-at-home women used to be supported by a tightly knit structure that might include mothers and mothers-in-law, aunts, sisters, cousins, and neighborhood women. They gave and received the support it took to maintain women's positive mental health.

In contrast, we modern women do not benefit from the luxury of a female support group. Telephone or e-mail communication just isn't as personal as a hug or a shared cup of coffee. Sisters are struggling to keep their own families intact. We don't really know our neighbors. We're isolated, alone, and emotionally impoverished.

Where Are You on the Economic Ladder?

Finances are another stressor. Even in the twenty-first century, women are likely to earn a lower salary than men for the same job and with the same qualifications. A stay-at-home mom, entirely dependent on her partner for income, may face poverty if her partner leaves or dies. But the financial inequality really hits single parents; among all the demographic groups, single mothers with dependent children have the highest rate of poverty.[13] According to the 2002 Health and Human Resources (HHS) Poverty Guidelines, a single mother with two children, with an income of $15,020 or less a year, is considered impoverished.[14]

Stress and Depression Go Hand-in-Hand

We women are stressed; our stress is making us depressed. One out of seven women will face a major depression sometime in her life. Women report twice the rate of depression compared to men.[15] Just being female sets us up for greater risk of depression.

Some depression is physiological. Hormone storms caused by imbalances among estrogen, progesterone, and testosterone may predispose us to physiological depression. Social influences may also set us up for a mood disorder.

Is It Real Depression—or a Bad Case of the Blues?

It is critical to distinguish between serious, clinical depression and garden-variety "blues." Sorrow, fear, anger, and guilt are all part of the human experience. Ordinary sadness is a rational response to disappointing life events. Women who are bearing the full responsibility of the family, in the absence of a supportive partner, can feel so overwhelmed by this burden that they sink into a state of chronic blues. Women who are not actively engaged in life, who do not enjoy challenging, fulfilling work, or whose lives are in constant chaos can begin to feel emotionally drained. Emotional exhaustion can "wear out" the adrenal gland, the symptoms of which can include the feeling that life is just too difficult to carry on. Exhaustion can feel very much like depression. Clinical depression, however, may be triggered by errant brain chemistry and/or unresolved psychological issues.

Depression can be exogenous (resulting from the loss of or separation from an important person or thing), or it can be endogenous (coming from within, usually severe, and without apparent cause). Both types of depression can be life threatening and require treatment.

WHAT IS DEPRESSION?

Depression is diagnosed by its duration and intensity, says Judy Hodel, M.S.W., C.I.S.W., a psychotherapist in Green Bay, Wisconsin. "If the person stops normal activities, if there's a change in eating and sleeping patterns, if there's a loss of interest in things usually of interest to the individual, if it lasts longer than two weeks, it's probably a major depression," says Hodel.[16] According to the American Psychiatric Association's Diagnostic and Statistical Manual of Mental Disorders, depression is defined by the following:

- Poor appetite and significant weight loss, or increased appetite and significant weight gain.
- Seasonal affective disorder normally occurs during the winter. It is most common in northern climates. Symptoms include low mood, poor motivation, lack of energy, and weight gain.
- Manic depression is also known as bipolar disorder. Symptoms usually emerge in the late teens and early adult life. The manic phase is characterized by hyperactivity, increased irritability, and reduced need for sleep. Symptoms of the depressive phase have already been described.

It's Not Just All in Our Heads

The roots of depression are by no means limited to social and emotional stressors. Our bodies are, by their physical nature, more prone to emotional disorders.

As we discussed in Chapter 3, hormonal havoc, as well as emotional havoc, are associated with puberty, premenstrual syndrome, and menopause. By-products of this hormonal turmoil include irritability, anxiety, depression, mood swings, difficulty concentrating, and lethargy, as well as weight gain, fluid retention, breast tenderness, joint or muscle pain, nausea, vomiting, and headaches. Women know very well how "mental" the symptoms of hormone imbalance really are. One of the first symptoms of impending menopause can be severe depression or other mood disorders.

Some of these hormone-related mood problems can begin at puberty, a time when gender distinctions in depression and other mood disorders may kick in. Before the onset of puberty, rates of depression among boys are as high, or even higher, than rates in girls. However, after puberty, girls are twice as likely to suffer from depression as are boys the same age.[17]

Gender distinctions in mood disorders continue throughout a woman's lifetime. From 10 to 15 percent of pregnant women experience depression, and as many as 80 percent suffer from the postpartum blues. When a history of mood disorders bumps up against a pregnancy or recent delivery, a woman's risk of depression is tripled. Postpartum psychosis, a more severe form of mental disorder, affects one out of a thousand women.

As women proceed through menopause, they often experience dark times of depression as hormone storms rage. Depression or anxiety disorders are often one of the first signs of approaching perimenopause.

Up to 35 percent of all women may exhibit signs of clinical or subclinical depression, rates that are far higher than those for men. Depression may be an early sign of thyroid dysfunction. Even slight decreases in thyroid hormone can generate depressive symptoms; however, it's still unclear whether depression triggers low thyroid function, or low thyroid function triggers depression.[18]

Circadian rhythms are the complex system that keeps sleep and activity in balance over a twenty-four-hour period. Depressed women are more likely to sleep excessively, compared to depressed men.[19] Could it be that women's circadian rhythms are more vulnerable to disruption?

Anxiety often accompanies depression. Up to 96 percent of depressed patients experience anxiety at the same time. More than two-thirds of people with a common anxiety disorder (obsessive-compulsive disorder) suffer from depression, too.[20]

Physical Implications

Like anxiety, depression can undermine the cardiovascular system and overall health. One reason is that it is more difficult for the hearts of depressed women to speed up and slow down as the body requires.[21] But there are other issues involving the heart and depression.

Researchers at the Duke University Medical Center analyzed data on more than 1,200 cardiac patients whose progress had been followed for approximately nineteen years. At the beginning of the study, the patients were evaluated for depression. At the end of the study, more patients with high scores for depression had died of coronary disease, compared to those with low scores for depression. The author of the study noted that the impact of negative affect seemed particularly strong in patients younger than age fifty.[22]

Am I Anxious or Depressed?

There is a difference between anxiety and depression, although in reality, the two often coexist or overlap. One can be anxious and depressed at the same time, or be anxious or depressed. It may be difficult at times to distinguish between these two mood disorders so that appropriate treatment can be obtained.

Anxiety disorders can be so disturbing that one may feel that his or her life is, literally, in jeopardy. It is difficult to forget the symptoms: "jitters," insomnia, knotted stomach, trembling, sweating, maybe even shortness of breath or racing heartbeat, especially if someone has experienced a true anxiety attack. Many people have raced to the emergency room at the hospital, convinced they were experiencing a heart attack, only to be sent home again dismissively: "It's only anxiety. Calm down." Calming down in the middle of a panic attack is virtually impossible. "Relax!" may be one of the most useless suggestions in the English language.

Anxiety means "a state of being uneasy, apprehensive, or worried about what may happen." By its very nature, life is uncertain, even chaotic at times. There is really little about life we can completely control. Anxiety may be unavoidable. In fact, anxiety—up to a certain point—serves a useful function. It releases adrenal hormones that sharpen our senses, tense our muscles, and ready the cardiovascular system for increased exertion. That physiological "fight-or-flight" response can lend an important edge that helps us present a livelier speech, take a better exam, or facilitate greater productivity.

A little anxiety can be helpful. A lot of anxiety is harmful. When anxiety is persistent, is out of proportion to the situation, or interferes with normal functioning, it becomes an anxiety disorder. People suffering from anxiety disorders live in psychological prisons of dread, fears, and emotional isolation. They often feel that they are having heart attacks.

At least 20 percent of patients who see their family doctors are suffering from "functionally significant anxiety."[23] According to the National Institute of Mental Health, anxiety disorders affect more than 23 million people across the United States, making it the most widespread mental illness in the nation.

Why Are Some People More Anxious Than Others?

It seems some people are born anxious. They cry when they leave the womb, they cry in their cribs, and they cry for no apparent reason. Tiny upsets in their personal environment send them into a tizzy of unhappiness that seems disproportionate to the offense. As they grow up, instead of growing out of their sensitivity, they become even more anxious as life events overwhelm their natural ability to maintain emotional homeostasis. One of the greatest triggers for the development of an anxiety disorder is a past history of abuse (emotional, physical, and/or sexual).

Psychiatrist and author Marilyn Kroplick, M.D., believes that childhood influences have an enormous impact on adult anxiety. "If there was a lot of anxiety during your childhood, and you had a parent who had an anxiety disorder, that, in itself, is likely to create some kind of chemical change within your own brain," she says. This chemical change predisposes an individual to anxiety. And as the research shows, women may be even more susceptible to anxiety disorders than are men.

IS IT ANXIETY OR A HEART ATTACK?

Diagnosing anxiety disorders and/or heart disease is best left to health care professionals. If you experience what you believe to be an anxiety or panic attack, get to a hospital immediately and obtain an accurate diagnosis—it could save your life. Women are especially likely to dismiss symptoms of heart disease with "it's all in my head . . . I'm just anxious today," and delay receiving life-saving treatment. It is not always easy for physicians to distinguish the symptoms of cardiovascular disease from anxiety disorders; it is even more difficult for we women to distinguish those symptoms in ourselves.

If one is suffering from symptoms of anxiety, it is important to rule out physical ailments that can mimic anxiety disorders. These include ischemic heart disease, mitral valve prolapse, arrhythmias, hyperthyroidism, hypoglycemia, menopause, premenstrual syndrome (PMS), nutritional deficiencies, asthma, chronic obstructive pulmonary disease, or intake of caffeine, alcohol, amphetamines, corticosteroids, illicit drugs, or other stimulants. As complicated as this picture is, no wonder that diagnosing anxiety disorders and/or heart disease can be so difficult.

Other factors can trigger anxiety:[24]

- Physiological imbalances; specifically, imbalances of certain neurotransmitters in the brain
- Major life stresses such as spousal abuse, death of a loved one, chronic illness, or financial difficulties
- Poor self-image
- Genetic factors

Dr. Felitti's work on sexual abuse victims, as well as other well-designed studies, confirm this opinion. From the research, it appears that when an individual is exposed to periods of great stress during childhood, an exaggerated cortisol response is triggered by relatively minor stressful events throughout life, predisposing an individual to lifelong anxiety and tension.

These people "fly off the handle" easily and overreact to the slightest provocation. Cortisol release or the stress reaction becomes a learned behavior, partially as a self-defense mechanism learned when they were children.

Physical Implications

We simply cannot separate the body from the mind. What happens to one inevitably affects the other. Anxiety is often triggered by stress, which activates the adrenal glands to unleash adrenaline. Adrenaline prepares the body for a "fight-or-flight" response, causing the heart to race, the blood pressure to increase, the blood sugar to be dysregulated, and the female hormone system to go awry.

The types of prolonged, unrelenting stress that twenty-first-century women face on a daily basis present a physical challenge to a body that was built in antiquity. Our bodies are simply not built to operate under unrelenting strain. Prolonged, anxiety-generating stress has been linked to high blood pressure, increased LDL cholesterol levels, and heart disease.[25]

Compounding the danger, women under stress often self-medicate with unhealthy habits. Stress pulls down energy production and availability, creating constant fatigue. When women awaken, they should feel well rested, eager to attend to the tasks of the day. But if they didn't sleep well, they simply do not have the energy to get up and face a busy day.

To get through the day, a woman may rely on coffee, sugar, soft drinks, and pasta. She may also resort to smoking, drinking, or taking drugs (legal or otherwise) in a desperate attempt to raise energy levels. Caffeine stimulates a cortisol response, further aggravating the risk of heart disease, and pseudofoods strip the body of the very nutrients needed to handle stress.

COUNT TO TEN

Extreme anger can also magnify the risk of a heart attack by triggering the "fight-or-flight" mode. As the temper flares, the body releases stress hormones that speed the heartbeat. Some blood vessels, such as those in the gut, constrict, increasing the danger. In the meantime, blood platelets become sticky, raising the odds of disastrous clotting.[26]

Drinking coffee to raise energy levels truly is "robbing Peter to pay Paul." At some point, "Peter" will simply refuse to give it up—the adrenal glands are now exhausted, and the woman is a prime candidate for a heart event. If women are going to be healthy and reduce their risk of heart disease, they must get a handle on their stress.

The Answers

We have just identified three major emotional and mental triggers for the development and progression of heart disease: depression, past sexual/emotional/physical abuse, and anxiety. They dovetail together, don't they? How are we going to solve these life issues? It is not enough to say, "Calm down," "Cheer up," "Forget about it," as people so often say when a woman describes her anxiety, depression, or history of abuse.

But even though we can't *think* or *reason* away our emotional situations, there are many positive steps we can take to improve our mental health and as a result, reduce our risk of heart disease.

Potential Remedies

Although we cannot control all the stressors in our lives, we can choose how to react, and how to cope. We can, believe it or not, take control of our stress and our health. If you are facing severe stress, depression, or anxiety attacks, take the following steps, one at a time, to reduce your risk of heart disease.

Restrict Sugar Intake White sugar can be called an "antinutrient." Refined sugar can generate anxiety symptoms. White sugar is essentially pure blood sugar; little processing by the liver is required to convert table sugar into blood sugar, so simple sugars are quickly released into the bloodstream. To handle this "sugar rush," the pancreas releases insulin, a hormone that helps transport glucose into the cells. When huge amounts of sugar are dumped rapidly into the bloodstream, the pancreas reacts wildly, sending large amounts of insulin into the bloodstream to pull excess sugar out of the blood before the brain and other organs are damaged. As a result, sugar levels plunge too low, sending the hapless victim into hypoglycemia or low blood sugar. Low blood sugar excites the adrenal gland into producing the stress hormone cortisol, which stimulates an increase in blood sugar. The cortisol rush is characterized by anxiety, "jitters," spaciness, anger, and confusion.

Avoid Food Additives Realizing the dangers of excessive sugar intake, some people have switched to using artificial sweeteners such as Aspartame

(NutraSweet™), or other synthetic flavor enhancers such as monosodium glutamate (MSG) and nitrates. Each of these synthetic products can elicit allergy- and anxiety-like symptoms. Aspartame alone is linked with rapid heartbeat, shallow breathing, anxiety, and dizziness.

Reduce Alcohol Intake Alcohol, as a simple sugar, can also trigger hypoglycemic symptoms. Furthermore, excess alcohol undermines the central nervous system. It also sabotages the liver's ability to detoxify other chemicals, including drugs, hormones such as estrogens, and pesticides. Toxic levels of these chemicals can build up in the body, making anxiety symptoms (and overall health) worse.

Restrict Caffeine Intake Coffee and other caffeine-containing products directly stimulate several arousal mechanisms in the body. Caffeine drains the body's stores of B vitamins and minerals such as potassium, calcium, magnesium, and sodium (each one of which are essential to heart function). Caffeine increases heart arrhythmias, heart rate, and diastolic blood pressure.

Reducing coffee consumption also tends to improve the mood, especially when sugar is also eliminated. While these two simple dietary changes do not resolve depression for everyone, depression improves significantly for many individuals.[27]

Breaking a caffeine addiction can be difficult for some people, especially people who use coffee as a "pick-me-up" in the morning. Breaking the coffee habit immediately can result in severe headaches, especially if one is trying to break the habit "cold turkey." Try to cut back to one cup a day. If you have been drinking several cups of coffee per day, eliminate one cup at a time to reduce withdrawal symptoms. As you are reducing the stimulants (coffee and sugar), simultaneously increase the amount of energy-producing foods such as fresh fruits and vegetables. Learn to enjoy herbal teas or other natural beverages.

Get Up and Get Moving! Consistent, vigorous physical activity is probably the best antianxiety agent ever invented. Exercise stretches the muscles, focuses one's attention, and promotes restful slumber. Aerobic excercises include running, swimming, walking briskly, aerobics classes, bicycling, cross-country skiing, or even strenuous housecleaning and yard work.

When we experience anxiety, our adrenal glands work overtime to pump out adrenaline. Exercise burns off the adrenaline that would otherwise exacerbate anxiety symptoms. In addition, physical activity triggers the release of hormones, such as endorphins, that function as natural opiates.

Weightlifting may also help regulate mood. In one study, thirty-six older women (mean age 68.5 years) were randomly assigned to a moderate-intensity strength training program, a high-intensity training regimen, and a control group. After 12 weeks, both weightlifting groups enjoyed improved muscle strength and body composition. As for mood changes, both groups reported feeling more positive. However, anxiety levels were significantly reduced in the moderate-intensity group.

The authors of the study conclude, "A moderate-intensity rather than high-intensity of training regimen may be more beneficial for sedentary older women to improve psychological health."[28]

Numerous studies have confirmed the benefits of physical exercise in reducing depression. You may not feel like it—but get out there and get moving! You will reduce anxiety, depression, and stress and improve your heart health.

Hope for Depression

Controlling severe depression can be overwhelmingly difficult. Depressed women simply do not have the mental or emotional energy to take charge of their mental and physical health. Yes, exercise and a good diet are extremely helpful in elevating the mood, but when you are too depressed to care, exercise and dietary changes are impossible to initiate.

The first thing to remember is that depression is a life-threatening illness that requires professional medical treatment. If you or someone you know is suffering from clinical depression, seek appropriate medical treatment immediately.

Having said that, there are some wonderful natural remedies for mild to moderate depression. Some can be used in conjunction with prescription medications; others should not be used concurrently with drug therapies. If there is any question, check with your physician.

- First, talk to someone! If you have experienced a major trauma—even if it dates back to early childhood—you need to address the cause. Successful therapy can protect against recurring depression.

Professional counseling can be extremely useful in digging into the real issues and presenting solutions.

- Do not be afraid to cry. Crying lets people know you need their help. In addition, tears carry away toxins generated by emotional shock. Allowing yourself to grieve appropriately by crying can be extremely cathartic and healing. Yes, big boys and big girls do cry.

- Getting by "with a little help from your friends" is always a good idea. The therapeutic benefits of social support are uncontested. As we said earlier in this chapter, women in our era and our culture have been snatched out of their natural, supportive environment of mothers, grandmothers, sisters, aunts, and female cousins. Social support is, however, extremely important, especially during times of stress and depression. If you do not have any close friends, make friendship a priority in your life. Loving companions will enrich your life.

  Husbands can be supportive during times of grief and depression, but let's face it: women need women. Make a friend!

- Get involved in a cause you love. Altruistic people are able to lose themselves in others. Working for a greater good can help block out depression, make us less aware of our own inadequacies, and help us overcome our personal problems.

- Adopt a pet. Pets alleviate loneliness, generate interactions between people, provide unconditional love, and even improve immune function.

- Practice good mental hygiene—learn how to think appropriate thoughts. Learned optimism is possible. Best-selling author Andrew Weil, M.D., suggests that disordered brain chemistry is not the root of negative thoughts, but rather, negative thoughts lead to disordered brain chemistry.

- Try acupuncture. This ancient Eastern therapy is believed to trigger the release of "feel-good" endorphins, which induce relaxation and relieve depression.

- Increase your intake of omega-3 fatty acids, either by eating more fish, or by taking fish oil or flaxseed oil supplements. Omega-3 oils appear to benefit those with depression or manic depression (bipolar disorder).

- Find out about SAMe. The human body constructs S-adenosyl-methionine (SAMe) from the amino acid methionine. It is found in protein-rich foods such as fish, meat, and dairy products. SAMe supplements are also available. SAMe is used to treat symptoms of depression, as well as osteoarthritis.

Deficiencies in magnesium and zinc are directly linked to depression, anxiety disorders, panic attacks, and other mood disorders. Well over 50 percent of the population is deficient in magnesium, and the same number may be deficient in zinc as well. Magnesium is found in dark green, leafy vegetables, and we don't eat many of those. Zinc is found in red meat and oysters, and we have reduced our consumption of red meat as well. The average American ingests about 150 to 200 mg of magnesium in the daily diet; the RDA is 300 mg. The average American receives about 4 to 6 mg of zinc in the daily diet; the RDA is 15 mg. Many nutritionists believe that more zinc may be needed to "fund" the thousands of enzymes for which zinc is essential.

Both magnesium and zinc depend on coenzymes like B complex vitamins. Women tend to be deficient in several of the B complex vitamins, and these nutrients should be taken together to provide maximum benefit to the body.

IS ALLERGY THE PROBLEM?

Certain foods can often trigger depression and/or anxiety and panic disorders. Two of the foods most commonly associated with mood disorders include wheat and dairy products. Wheat often triggers mental symptoms such as mild to severe depression, confusion, anxiety, inappropriate sleepiness, and others.

Dairy products can also trigger mental symptoms, but any food can be an allergen. If you feel that your mood disorder may be associated with a food you are eating, eliminate the food for at least six weeks and see if your mood doesn't improve. Or, seek the counsel of a nutritionally trained physician who can help you diagnose your allergies or food intolerances.

An Herb for Depression

Some terrific studies on the use of St. John's wort, spanning several decades, have shown that this beautiful yellow flower can help to reduce the symptoms of mild to moderate depression. Millions of people have improved their own moods by using this herb.

St. John's wort is not a panacea; it does not produce significant benefits in everyone, because the root of depression is not the same in everyone. Some depression is biochemical in nature, and scientists believe that St. John's wort may work on the serotonergic pathways or other biochemical pathways in the brain.

This herb is best used in conjunction with nutrients such as magnesium, zinc, and the B-complex vitamins to guarantee that the body's nutritional needs are being met.

Solving the Mental/ Emotional Equation

It is no accident that the poetic heart is so inextricably linked to the physical heart. We really do, in many cases, carry our "hearts on our sleeves." We are emotional creatures; we needn't apologize for that.

By the same token, if we wish to care for our physical hearts, we must give thought to our "emotional hearts." We must heal our inner selves. Possibly one of the most healing of all practices is the practice of forgiveness. It seems that very few women escaped from childhood wholly intact emotionally.

One evening, in the middle of a course on health and weight management, a group of older women began talking about their personal "mother hunger." The discussion became very intimate as woman after woman began sharing the story of her relationship with her mother and how it had affected her throughout life. Some women had enjoyed nurturing, enriching relationships with their mothers; others had endured years of abuse at the hands of their mothers.

All had a "hunger" for their mothers, either for their real mothers who had since passed away, or for the mother they had all wished they had. The discussion came around to the importance of forgiveness. Those women who were able to release their anger and truly forgive their mothers (and others) who had injured them were healthy and strong. They had passed on a better heritage to their children.

Perhaps this is where we all need to go to find healing for our hearts. We can come to a place of releasing our hurts and letting them go. Lack of forgiveness is a terrible stress on the heart. Forgiveness is a soothing balm that heals and restores—even the heart.

CHAPTER 5

What Is a Healthy Diet, Anyway?

Back in the early days of the natural health movement, the role of diet and health was pooh-poohed vigorously. Nutrition was considered a "soft science." Medicine was "hard science." The hard science people did not respect the soft science people, and unfortunately, hard science took the forefront in research and medical practice. Drugs became the treatment of choice, not food.

Today, however, there is virtually no controversy about whether food can either heal or hurt the heart. We know that diet plays an integral role in the health of the heart and the rest of the body. The trick is to figure out just how—and which—diet influences health. What is a healthy diet? Is it low fat? High carbohydrate? Or high protein? What is natural food? We might be more compliant with dietary recommendations if they just stopped changing them!

Let's look at what the studies say. In the Nurses' Health Study, researchers studied food-frequency questionnaires from 69,017 women. These women ranged from ages thirty-eight to sixty-three. The researchers identified two major dietary patterns: the "prudent" diet and the "Western" diet. The prudent diet (a more traditional diet) was rich in fruits, vegetables, legumes (beans, lentils, peas), fish, poultry, and whole grains. The Western diet (what we *really* eat) emphasized red and processed meats, sweets and desserts, French fries, and refined grains.

After twelve years, 821 women had been diagnosed with coronary heart disease. After adjusting for coronary risk factors, the researchers found that the women who had consumed the prudent diet had a lower risk of coronary heart disease than those who had followed the Western diet.[1]

Now, here is just how crazy science gets. A group of cardiologists did a small study to test whether eating a plate of fresh fruits and veggies before a meal would influence serum cholesterol. Their conclusions? The authors feel that fruits and vegetables may be a safe adjunct to the prudent diet in high-risk individuals who need to lower their cholesterol and triglyceride levels and for prevention of coronary artery disease. (The diet included fruits and vegetables such as guava, grapes, papaya, bananas, sweet limes, oranges, apples, leaves of fenugreek, spinach, mustard, radishes, tomatoes, lotus root, bitter gourds, mushrooms, onions, garlic and trichosanthes, fenugreek seeds, grains, peas, kidney and red beans, and nuts such as almonds and walnuts.)[2]

Did you get that? They feel it *may* be a *safe adjunct*. Since when would fresh fruits and veggies be an unsafe adjunct to any diet? Do we really need to study that? It is a sad state when doctors are reluctant to put their unqualified stamp of approval on bananas, onions, and spinach.

Thousands of studies over the past several decades point to the inevitable conclusion that a traditional diet (in whatever form that may take) is good for the heart. It is only when we start tampering with the food supply, creating pseudofoods that we run into trouble.

Why Do So Many Women Struggle with Obesity?

The jury is in. The modern Western diet is a key culprit in the rising rate of obesity. We know that excess weight is a primary risk factor for heart disease. In fact, the American Heart Association recognizes that obesity is a major modifiable factor for coronary heart disease. Obesity is an influence on high total cholesterol levels, high triglyceride levels, and low HDL cholesterol levels. Gaining only 1 pound of fat a year can gradually increase total cholesterol and reduce HDL cholesterol.[3]

In addition, excess body fat increases the level of insulin in the blood. High insulin levels are associated with sodium and water retention—two contributing factors in hypertension. Furthermore, excess weight can speed the heart rate and slow the capacity of blood vessels to transport blood. These factors also raise blood pressure.

Obesity increases susceptibility to stroke. Obesity, and the dietary elements that contribute to excess weight, may lead to a buildup of fatty deposits in arteries, including the arteries in the brain. If a blood clot develops in a constricted artery in the brain, blood flow to that area of the brain is blocked, causing stroke.

Health providers are encouraged to work with their patients on obesity management. But here again, we run into no small amount of trouble. Losing weight is much easier to discuss than to do. That is especially true for women.

Yes, it is more difficult for women to lose weight than for men, and it is easier for us to gain weight. When men undertake a sensible weight loss program, they can expect to lose 2 pounds a week. When women try to lose weight, they only lose, on average, 1 pound a week, and often not even that.

Upper body fat is associated with Syndrome X, a cluster of symptoms including high cholesterol, unbalanced HDL/LDL levels, high triglycerides, high circulating insulin levels, and excess weight, particularly in the abdominal and upper body regions. Lower-body fat (in the hips and thighs) is associated with hormone imbalance and will not easily be lost by diet alone.

There are some very important physiological reasons for added weight gain in women. Even those issues that we consider to be psychological, or embedded deep within the woman's psyche, are driven by hormones. In other words, women, your fat is not your fault!

Let's look at these physiological issues, one by one, to help relieve women's dietary guilt—and save their hearts.

1. Women have far more estrogen than testosterone. This fact influences added fat weight and lower muscle weight. Women do not produce much testosterone, a "male" hormone that increases metabolism, directs the body to lay down more muscle tissue, and lightens the fat load.

When women become estrogen dominant (hormones between estrogen and progesterone are unbalanced), weight management becomes even more difficult. Progesterone deficiency leads to lowered metabolism, increased chocolate and/or sugar cravings, lowered body temperature, fatigue, depression, and other conditions that drive eating behaviors and reduce the number of calories burned.

Because women do not produce much testosterone, it is more difficult for them to lay down lean muscle mass, even if they do a vigorous workout at the gym.

2. The menstrual cycle can lead to excess weight. The natural female cycle begins on day one (the first day of menses), with an increase in estrogen. Estrogen is dominant for the first fourteen days of the cycle, called the fol-

licular stage. Around day seven, estrogen begins to wane. By day fifteen, progesterone levels begin to rise, reaching their highest level about day twenty-one. During this stage, the luteal stage, the body is preparing for pregnancy. Because pregnancy places additional demands on the body, other physiological changes begin to occur.

For example, the body's metabolic rate begins to increase, and there is an increased demand for calories to meet the higher metabolic demands. So, unfortunately, while women tend to burn more calories the last half of the cycle, they also tend to eat more calories, primarily in the form of sweets.

Because the body anticipates pregnancy, additional water stores are laid down (water retention).Women frequently gain 5 or more pounds of excess water at this time, only to lose it after the start of the period.

Few of us experience a truly normal menstrual cycle, however, and the cycle often adds unwanted weight. For example, the environment is becoming increasingly burdened with xenoestrogens that act as estrogen mimics or estrogen blockers. Many of us remain estrogen dominant throughout the cycle, a condition that leads to enhanced fat deposition, increased stress on the thyroid (causing hypothyroidism), and lowered levels of testosterone.

How significant is the premenses caloric increase? Carbohydrate intake from meals increases by as much as 24 percent, and as much as 43 percent from snacks. Most of the increases are in the form of refined carbohydrates and fat.

3. The week before the onset of menstruation, the calming mineral magnesium is burned more rapidly, producing cravings for chocolate and sweets and contributing to depression, fatigue, muscle cramps, and many other unpleasant symptoms. The list of magnesium-deficiency symptoms nearly duplicates the list of PMS or menopause symptoms. In other words, PMS and menopause may actually be a "symptom" of magnesium deficiency rather than a true syndrome.

4. Most women are tired nearly all the time! Many are holding down at least two full-time jobs: homemaker and out-of-the-home worker. To keep up with the demands of both, women self-medicate with coffee, sugar, and soft drinks, which only makes their weight and health profile more fragile.

Caffeine increases the production of cortisol, which hastens the breakdown of lean muscle tissue, causes memory loss, and increases fat deposition, primarily in the abdomen and waist. Stress itself causes excess fat in the middle region; caffeine only accentuates the problem.

Stress eating is common. Stress eaters may reach for sugars (in an attempt to deal with their accompanying fatigue), or salty, crunchy foods. Salt helps shore up flagging energy stores, increases water retention, adding to upper-body weight. It also throws off blood sugar levels, thereby triggering harmful eating behaviors.

5. Women do not get enough sleep! The average American woman is sleep deprived by more than one hour per night, leading to constant grogginess or fatigue. To mask their exhaustion, many women self-medicate with coffee.

Add these up: Imbalance between estrogen and progesterone, lower production of testosterone, stress, sleep deprivation, and—oh yes, let's not forget depression, another major trigger for weight problems. Depression has also been linked to overweight due to an increase in poor eating habits (binging on chocolate, sweets, or other stimulants) and/or use of antidepressant medications.

Depression can be caused by many factors, including psychological problems, hypothyroidism, hypoadrenalism, food allergies, chemical imbalances, toxic metal accumulation, nutrient deficiencies, or other physical/nutritional disorders. It can also be caused by low levels of serotonin and/or dopamine, or imbalances between the catecholamines. (Catecholamines are a family of nitrogen-containing compounds derived from the amino acid tyrosine.) Whatever triggers it, depression can lead to eating behaviors that may reflect the body's attempt to elevate the mood. Depression itself often triggers cravings for carbohydrates.

Are you convinced yet? Most women do not need to be told about the difficulty of losing weight; they have been frustrated for a long time about that very issue.

Now that we understand why we eat the things we do, let's discuss what we *should* eat. First, let's see what the experts say.

Dietary Guidelines Set by the Experts

The following diets have been widely publicized, and they have all helped women and men boost their heart health. Can we make sense of the research? After reading the studies, can we actually prepare a meal without feeling frustrated?

If anyone should know what a healthy diet is, it should be the American

Heart Association. The AHA has designed two types of diets, one for prevention and one to help treat heart disease.

The American Heart Association (AHA) Diet

The AHA diet includes Steps 1 and 2. The Step 1 diet is designed for people who do not have heart disease but want to prevent it. It recommends a daily fat intake of no more than 30 percent of total calories. Saturated fats should comprise only 10 percent of the diet. In the Step 1 diet, 50 to 65 percent of total calories should come from complex carbohydrates.

The Step 2 diet addresses people who already have heart disease or high cholesterol levels. In this diet, fat makes up only 20 percent of total calories, and saturated fat, only 7 percent. The Step 2 diet recommends a dietary cholesterol intake of less than 200 mg daily.[4]

Research suggests that the benefits of the AHA diet are modest. One study examined the impact of reduced fat and saturated fat intake on cholesterol levels. At the end of eight weeks, study participants demonstrated lower levels of HDL "good" cholesterol.[5] In other words, the diet did not significantly improve the important HDL/LDL ratio.

The Mediterranean Diet

The Mediterranean diet is certainly more pleasurable. It emphasizes whole grains, fish, olive oil, garlic, and moderate consumption of red wine. Thirty-five to 45 percent of total calories come from fat. However, these are monounsaturated and polyunsaturated fats. Mary Flynn, Ph.D., coauthor of *Low-Fat Lies, High-Fat Frauds* (Lifeline Press, 1999) says, "Countries consuming olive oil, even in high amounts, have lower rates of chronic diseases such as heart disease, certain cancers, osteoporosis, cataracts, arthritis, gallbladder disease, hypertension, and stroke."[6]

Fish is the primary protein source. The Mediterranean diet also includes more fresh fruits and vegetables, nuts, and legumes than are found in the standard American diet.

One review focused on olive oil, a staple of the Mediterranean diet. The authors of the review pointed out that olive oil increases plasma levels of HDL cholesterol and decreases LDL cholesterol. As an antioxidant, olive oil protects against lipid peroxidation, a risk factor in atherosclerosis and heart disease.

Red wine is also an integral part of the Mediterranean diet. A rich source of antioxidants, red wine protects cholesterol against oxidation. The authors of one study concluded, "Our data indicate that red wine components bind to LDL and HDL and protect these lipoproteins from . . . lipid peroxidation."[7] Some research suggests that purple grape juice exerts comparable benefits.

The Mediterranean diet is relatively low in iron and calcium. If you choose to follow this diet, consider taking supplemental calcium. If you're a premenopausal woman, and your iron levels are low, talk to your doctor about iron supplements.

The Ornish Program

The diet developed by Dean Ornish, M.D., targets individuals who have cholesterol problems, but do not want to, or cannot, take cholesterol-lowering drugs. This is a difficult diet to follow. The Ornish program prohibits all oils, animal products (except for egg whites), nonfat milk, and nonfat yogurt. In this program, total fats make up 10 percent of daily calories, and complex carbohydrates make up 75 percent.

Because it is a low-calorie eating plan, the Ornish program usually results in weight loss. When overweight people slim down, they reduce their risk of heart disease.

A controlled trial investigated the long-term effects of the Ornish program. Twenty-eight women and men, whose arteries were partially blocked, followed the program for one year. At the end of the year, patients on the Ornish program experienced a 91 percent decrease in the frequency of angina, a 42 percent decrease in the duration of angina, and a 28 percent decrease in the severity of angina. In contrast, the control group demonstrated a 165 percent increase in frequency, a 95 percent increase in duration, and a 39 percent increase in severity of angina.

Ornish states, "While moderate reductions in dietary fat and cholesterol have little effect on plasma LDL cholesterol, more substantial reductions may cause reductions in LDL cholesterol comparable to cholesterol-lowering drugs."[8]

The problem with the Ornish plan is that it is seriously deficient in a number of nutrients, including essential fatty acids, fat-soluble vitamins A and E, folic acid (needed to lower homocysteine levels), calcium, iron, and zinc. The other problem is hunger and noncompliance. It is virtually impossible to defeat hunger indefinitely, as hunger is a necessary body communication tool to prevent people from willingly starving to death.

One benefit of the Ornish program is that one can eat as much as one wants—as long as it is a vegetable or a grain. There is no question that, in the short term, the Ornish program works to lower the risk factors for heart disease. The problem is long-term malnutrition. A program that doesn't provide the fundamental base of nutrition is not a lifetime solution.

Dietary Approaches to Stop Hypertension (DASH)

The DASH diet emphasizes whole grains, fruits, vegetables, and low-fat dairy products and includes very little saturated fat or sodium. The DASH diet include nuts, seeds, legumes, and moderate amounts of lean protein from fish, poultry, or soy foods. The DASH diet contains two-and-a-half times the levels of potassium, calcium, and magnesium found in the standard American diet.[9]

One study explored the impact of the DASH diet on seventy-two people with stage 1 hypertension. After eight weeks on the DASH diet, 78 percent of the study participants lowered their systolic blood pressure. The authors of the study report, "Our results indicate that the DASH diet . . . is effective as first-line therapy in stage 1 isolated systolic hypertension."[10]

At least one study suggests that the DASH approach may affect cholesterol levels. For eight weeks, some of the study participants followed the DASH diet. At the end of the study, the DASH group demonstrated a greater reduction in total cholesterol levels than did the control group.[11]

The DASH program emphasizes fresh, whole foods. As a result, the diet is rich in nutrients needed to protect the heart, such as potassium, calcium, and magnesium.

Best Foods for Heart Health

Food can be your medicine or your poison. Before we go into the details about what you should prepare for dinner tonight, let's review some of the foods that are most beneficial to the heart. How do these foods help prevent heart disease—or reverse it once the process has already started?

Some of the best heart-friendly foods available include the following.

Fish

Fish provides a wealth of omega-3 fatty acids, "good" fats that support heart health. Fish that contain high levels of omega-3 oils include salmon, mackerel, sardines, herring, anchovies, whitefish, and bluefish.

Fish or fish oil may effectively thin the blood, thereby protecting against blood clots. It also appears to reduce high blood pressure and improve insulin sensitivity, which indirectly affects heart health. A prospective study explored the relationship between fish intake and the risk of stroke in women. Researchers looked at 79,839 women from the Nurses' Health Study cohort. In 1980, when the study started, the participants ranged from ages thirty-four to fifty-nine. None had been diagnosed with heart disease, cancer, diabetes, or high total cholesterol levels.

After fourteen years, 574 strokes were reported. The researchers discovered that women who ate fish two or more times a week had a reduced risk of total stroke and thrombotic infarction (stroke caused by blood clot). The authors of the study conclude, "Our data indicate that higher consumption of fish and omega-3 polyunsaturated fatty acids is associated with a reduced risk of thrombotic infarction, primarily among women who do not take aspirin regularly."[12]

Fish oils are anti-inflammatory, help reduce blood clotting, help maintain a healthy HDL/LDL level, and confer many other benefits to the body. The benefits of omega-3 oils are discussed further in Chapter 6.

The Mercury Question When the benefits of fish are discussed, another question frequently arises: "What about the mercury in ocean-raised fish? Are farm-raised fish safer?"

This is an important and difficult issue. We live in a very polluted environment. The oceans of our world contain dangerous levels of toxic substances, like mercury, that work their way up through the food chain. The seafood that we enjoy contains heavy metals and other poisons that embed themselves in our tissues. Mercury is one of the most toxic substances on the planet, and it lays down into nerve tissue, wreaking havoc throughout the body.

The problem with farm-raised fish, however, is that growers do not supply the fish with their own natural foods. Moreover, the fish are often not exposed to the same climatic conditions as wild fish, so their bodies do not produce the same amount of omega-3 fats. Even if the farm-raised fish is safer in terms of toxic metals, it does not provide the same high level of nutrition as wild fish.

Much of the seafood available in American supermarkets is farm raised; some is wild. It is difficult to know where seafood comes from. Many nutritionists believe that organic seafood should be chosen whenever possible. By all means, avoid eating any type of seafood that has been grown in openly polluted waters, such as the ocean surrounding Indonesia.

It is a good policy to get your toxic metal load checked from time to time. Consider hair analysis, or packed erythrocyte testing, performed by a competent laboratory. These diagnostic tools can provide valuable information about the toxic metal load of the body and can provide you some direction on how to chelate these metals out of the system.

We should all question whether our seafood provides the levels of omega-3 fatty acids that our hearts require. Using organic, toxin-free fish oil capsules can provide some insurance about the quality of our fatty acid intake.

Fruits

Fruits are rich in fiber and antioxidants—two important heart protectors. Water-soluble fiber has been shown to lower cholesterol. Apparently, it helps produce a gel in the intestines that attaches to cholesterol and sweeps it out of the body. In addition, fiber-rich foods such as fruit satisfy the human appetite for sweets. The most fiber-rich fruits include apples, pears, strawberries, prunes, oranges, and bananas.

Antioxidants in fruit help prevent the oxidation of LDL cholesterol. Although we need oxygen to stay alive, oxidation can also be harmful to our health. For example, it can transform LDL into damaging, plaque-forming material. Vitamins C and E and carotenoids, specifically, are known to ward off oxidative, or free radical destruction.

Vegetables

Like fruit, vegetables are rich in minerals, fiber, and antioxidants. It is no accident that vegetarians have lower rates of cardiovascular disease and hypertension, as well as diabetes and some cancers. They also typically have lower blood pressure and lower heart disease mortality rates than the general population.

Vegetables are nature's own mineral supplement. Vegetables that are grown in good soil, picked when ripe, and eaten while still fresh and minimally cooked provide a rich source of minerals. These include potassium, magnesium, calcium, and other trace minerals, all of which are beneficial to the heart.

Vegetables contain lots of fiber. The cell membrane of vegetables contains fibrous material that is indigestible in the human digestive tract. This fiber "sweeps" the intestinal tract clean as it passes through the small and large intestines. Fiber provides a haven for friendly bacteria, symbiotic organisms that provide many benefits to human health. Fiber helps clear excess cholesterol out of the large intestine before it can be reabsorbed and lead to higher serum cholesterol.

Vegetables provide thousands of bioflavonoids, nutrients with benefits that scientists are still discovering. Some of those benefits confer antioxidant protection, but bioflavonoids protect the human body in other ways, too.

The most nutrient-packed vegetables are deeply colored. Choose dark green garden lettuce, for example, over iceberg. Broccoli is preferable to cauliflower, although both provide impressive nutritional clout.

Furthermore, vegetables provide B vitamins. These nutrients can help prevent high homocysteine levels, which are implicated in heart disease. (See Chapter 6 for more information about homocysteine.)

Raw, fresh vegetables may be a better choice, overall, than cooked vegetables. Typically, raw vegetables contain higher concentrations of nutrients than cooked ones. They also contain enzymes, specialized proteins that can thin the blood, protect against blood clots, and reduce arterial plaque. Cooking can deplete vegetables of their nutritional value. If you decide to cook your vegetables, lightly steam them, and do not overcook them.

Legumes

Legumes include beans, lentils, and peas. An abundance of fiber, amino acids, iron, B vitamins, and calcium is available from legumes. Calcium is known to promote optimal blood pressure. People who eat legume-rich diets are more likely to have healthy cholesterol levels. Legumes are a mainstay of vegetarian diets because they supply many of the same nutrients that meat does, including iron, protein, and B vitamins.

The most health-promoting legumes include dry beans such as French, kidney, navy, snap, stringless, and green beans; adzuki beans; alfalfa sprouts; carob; chickpeas; fava beans; lentils; lima beans; mung beans; peas; string beans, and possibly soybeans.

Whole Grains

Whole grains, especially oats, are frequently recommended for the heart and overall health. The most widely used food grains include oats, wheat, rice, and corn. Whole grains are found in breakfast cereals, pasta, and bread. These low-calorie foods are packed with fiber and complex carbohydrates. Whole grains include barley, rice, buckwheat (kasha), millet, oats, quinoa, bulgur, and cracked wheat.

Oats, along with nuts, are particularly good for the heart. A study funded by Quaker Oats at Tufts University in Boston investigated forty-three women and men who ate a diet rich in oats. At the end of the six-week study, the participants demonstrated lower blood pressure and cholesterol.[13]

Another study, also funded by Quaker Oats, suggests that oatmeal can protect against the damaging impact of a high-fat diet. Specifically, it may prevent decreased blood flow, a sign of endothelial dysfunction, which is errant blood vessel behavior.[14] People with heart disease, or risk factors for heart disease, often experience endothelial dysfunction. However, healthy individuals may also experience endothelial dysfunction after eating a high-fat meal.

In 1997, the Food and Drug Administration (FDA) authorized the use of a specific health claim on the label for whole oats, oat bran, rolled oats, and whole oat flour. The decision was based on the ability of water-soluble fiber from whole oats to reduce total cholesterol levels.

There is controversy, however, about the role of grains, specifically wheat, in a heart-healthy diet. In individuals who are insulin resistant or carbohydrate sensitive, eating ground grains can elevate insulin levels and increase insulin resistance. In one study, researchers tested several types of meals on blood glucose and plasma insulin levels. They found that eating foods made from ground grains (flour products) raised blood sugar and insulin levels 30, 60, 90, 120, 180, and 240 minutes after the meal, as opposed to meals without grain products. Sticky rice also elevated insulin levels. The meals with higher insulin responses also tended to cause higher C-peptide responses, another risk factor for the development of heart disease.[15]

This study was done with a diabetic population. Another study on diabetes suggests that wheat, soy, and to a lesser degree, milk, may actually *lead* to the development of diabetes mellitus, particularly when these foods are introduced early in life.

A synopsis of this article reads:

WHOLE-GRAIN CAVEATS

Do not be fooled by fluffy supermarket breads that are labeled "wheat" and are brown in color. The color is not typically from rich, brown grain; the color comes from molasses or another coloring agent. It is impossible to make a fluffy, whole-wheat loaf. Whole wheat naturally contains lots of fiber that makes a true, whole-grain bread dense and firm. Be sure to read the label; if it lists "enriched flour" it is *not* a whole-grain bread. If possible, purchase your whole-grain breads from a whole-food supermarket that maintains high standards of nutritional quality.

> Insulin-dependent diabetes mellitus is very likely to be initiated by food containing diabetogens such as wheat, soy, and to a lesser degree, cow's milk, given early on in life. Insulin-dependent diabetes mellitus may be prevented or delayed by avoiding these foods until weaning, or even as late as adolescence. . . . Most diabetes cases require long-term food exposure to diabetogens after infancy; the time around puberty is particularly important. The probability of preventing diabetes by avoiding only one dietary diabetogen in the first six months of life is small. Diet appears to have a major effect on both target cells and attacking leukocytes.[16]

This information is troubling indeed, especially for individuals who are consciously trying to sort through the confusing, misleading data and make sense of it. Does wheat improve heart health—or contribute to heart disease via the development of diabetes? What about other grains? Which ones are problematic?

Wheat is categorized as one of the top three allergens in the world. An amazing variety of health problems can often be linked to wheat allergy or wheat intolerance.

There is not a lot of research on this issue, but prudence may suggest eliminating wheat as a significant source of nutrition, particularly if an individual has a family or personal history of diabetes or other blood sugar problems.

Soy Products

Soy is a legume as well as a dietary supplement. This versatile food helps lower cholesterol, thereby lowering the risk of atherosclerosis and heart disease.

Here again, controversy arises about the benefits of, or harm from, consuming soy products. While many studies have indeed shown some benefits from using soy as a protein source, other information points to potential problems with soy. These include hypothyroidism, food allergy, blocked absorption of minerals, and increased estrogen dominance. Soy will be discussed in more detail in Chapter 6.

Nuts

Nuts are certainly not a low-calorie food. Some women and men avoid eating them because of their high fat content. However, nuts contain monounsaturated fats, which are known to lower LDL cholesterol levels. Walnuts are especially high in linolenic acid, a polyunsaturated fatty acid. Linolenic acid demonstrates an anticlotting effect.

One Harvard study involved 86,000 women from the Nurses' Health Study. Researchers found that women who ate 1 ounce (about ¼ cup) of nuts per day had a 35 percent lower risk of heart disease.[17] A crossover study focused on macadamia nuts. Thirty volunteers followed three, 30-day diets in random order: the standard American diet (SAD), comprised of 37 percent fat; the AHA Step 1 diet; and a macadamia nut-based monounsaturated fat diet. Lower total cholesterol levels were noted after the AHA and macadamia nut–based diets. Not surprisingly, cholesterol levels after the SAD were higher.[18]

The Worst Foods for Heart Health

Some "experts" are known for the mantra, "There is no such thing as a bad food." That is nonsense! In our pathological American food culture, the supermarket shelves are lined with pseudofoods that damage the heart, poison the brain, and cause many degenerative diseases.

As we explore diet, it will be instructive to investigate the world of "bad nutrition." Let's get these harmful products out of our kitchens and out of our bodies. By limiting or avoiding the following foods or food components, you may reduce your risk of high cholesterol, high blood pressure, heart disease, and possibly premature death.

Bad Fats

Trans-fatty acids and excessive amounts of saturated fats are two of your heart's worst enemies. Saturated fats become solid at room temperature. Stores of these fats can build up in the arteries and thereby slow down blood flow. Saturated fats are present in meats, poultry, eggs, butter, cheese, whole milk, and cream. Unfortunately, the standard American diet includes high amounts of these foods.

It is not a good idea to eliminate all saturated fats, however. Saturated fats were included in the traditional diet because they are essential to human health. The problem is that we consume too much of these types of fats and are deficient in unsaturated fats that provide fatty-acid balance.

To reduce your consumption of saturated fat, reduce your intake of poultry with skin, butter, and whole milk or whole-milk foods.

Trans-fatty acids are even worse. Also known as hydrogenated fats, trans-fatty acids may increase LDL cholesterol and heighten your risk of heart disease. If you want to reduce your intake of trans-fatty acids, cut down on fried foods and use oils or tub margarine instead of stick margarine. Even better, replace margarine with a small amount of butter. If you are concerned that you are still eating too much saturated fat, mix softened butter half-in-half with olive oil. Olive oil is rich in monounsaturated fats that are protective of the heart—and it tastes good, too!

A study on saturated fats and trans-fatty acids focused on their impact on 80,082 women from the Nurses' Health Study. When the study started in 1980, the women were between thirty-four to fifty-nine years old. At that time, they had no diagnosed heart disease, stroke, high cholesterol levels, diabetes, or cancer. Researchers obtained information on their diets, and followed up with food questionnaires.

After fourteen years, researchers documented 939 cases of nonfatal heart attack and deaths from heart disease. After examining the dietary information, they concluded that every 5 percent reduction in saturated fat equaled a 42 percent drop in heart disease risk. Every 2 percent reduction in trans-fatty acids equaled a 53 percent drop in risk.

As we discussed before, not all fats are bad. The authors of the above-cited study state, "Our findings suggest that replacing saturated and trans-unsaturated fats with unhydrogenated monounsaturated and polyunsaturated fats is more effective in preventing heart disease in women than reducing overall fat intake."[19]

Unhydrogenated monounsaturated fats are found in olive, peanut, canola, avocado, and some fish oils. These benign fats are believed to lower cholesterol levels. Polyunsaturated fats are available in sesame, safflower, and sunflower oils. Omega-3 fatty acids are one type of polyunsaturated fat. Omega-3s are found in tuna, mackerel, salmon, and other fatty fish. They protect against blood clots, as well as atherosclerosis.

One must be careful when evaluating information about various types of fats. Not all fats are equal in terms of heart health. Numerous studies compare fish oil with corn oil, for example. The majority of the studies indicate that fish oil lowers serum cholesterol, helps balance the HDL/LDL cholesterol fraction, lowers triglycerides, and provides anti-inflammatory protection, whereas corn oil does not. (Keep in mind that corn is one of the top three allergens in the world.)

Fat is an incredibly fragile nutrient, prone to rancidity on exposure to oxygen and light. Therefore, the only fats that should be considered "good food" are fats that are minimally processed and as fresh as possible. For example, olive oil should be purchased in small quantities and used quickly. If canola oil is chosen, purchase only cold-pressed, raw canola oil, keep it refrigerated, and use it as quickly as possible. Butter should be kept refrigerated; raw nuts and seeds should be kept refrigerated and used quickly before the fats turn rancid; and so on.

Processed fats (especially heat-processed, hydrogenated food products) should be strictly avoided. There is some indication that consuming hydrogenated oils blocks the absorption of beneficial oils, increasing the possibility of a deficiency of "good" fats.

Beef

Beef is certainly a mainstay of the standard American diet. Some restaurants advertise 16- or even 24-ounce steaks. As the advertisements say, "Beef. It's what's for dinner."

Why would anyone want (or need) to eat a 24-ounce steak? One can almost see the cholesterol clogging up the arteries after a gluttonous meal of 16- or 24-ounce steaks, baked potato stuffed with butter and sour cream, broccoli with cheese sauce, salad with gooey dressing, and a bowl of ice cream for dessert. It might be wise for most restaurants to keep a cardiologist on staff just to deal with the heart attacks waiting in the wings after these types of meals!

Although we may love our steak, ribs, and hamburgers, they don't love us. While we cannot assume that meat restriction is the sole reason for the lower rates of coronary heart disease among Mediterranean populations, we can glean some valuable information from this epidemiological data. The Mediterranean diet also provides a wealth of fruit, vegetables, and whole grains. In addition, the Mediterranean diet emphasizes the use of olive oil, a balance between the saturated and unsaturated fats, and a balance of omega-3 to omega-6 fatty acids.

Beef isn't all bad. It supplies iron, protein, zinc, selenium, and B vitamins. Coenzyme Q10 and L-carnitine are also to be found in beef. On the other hand, these valuable nutrients are also available in other foods, as well as in dietary supplements. So, if you do choose to eat beef, make your beef portions small, and when possible, organic.

Sodium

Sodium restriction is usually recommended for people with hypertension, although there is some speculation that only sodium-sensitive individuals need to cut down.

The twelve-week DASH–Sodium Study involved 412 individuals. For the first four weeks, participants consumed about 3,300 mg of salt—the average salt intake in the standard American diet. In the next four weeks, they consumed about 2,400 mg daily. In the final four weeks, the subjects reduced their salt intake to 1,500 mg daily. The results were impressive. The less salt these individuals consumed, the more their blood pressure dropped. People with hypertension saw the most benefit: their systolic blood pressure dropped an average of 11.5 points.[20]

Claude Lenfant, M.D., former director of the National Heart, Lung, and Blood Institute (NHLBI), states, "These findings show that a [salt] intake below that now recommended could help many Americans prevent the blood pressure rises that now occur with advancing age."

The National Research Council of the National Academy of Sciences concurs. This group has reported that the ideal sodium level is around 1,800 milligrams a day. The standard American diet includes twice that much.

Sodium is found in table salt, bologna, hot dogs, tomato ketchup, cold breakfast cereal, pickled foods, and salad dressing. Sodium is also found in milk shakes, cheese, canned soups, baked goods, baking soda, and even cow's milk. Furthermore, laxatives and antacids contain high levels of sodium. Check food labels very carefully for sodium content.

The twenty-first-century supermarket frozen food aisle presents a bewildering variety of packaged, frozen entrees with such misnomers as "Healthy Choice" or "Lean Cuisine." The picture on the front of the box is more appetizing than the contents.

Turn the package over and read the nutritional information on the back. The sodium content of these quick meals is staggering, ranging anywhere from 800 to more than 2,000 mg per serving. Some packages boast a fairly low sodium content (600 to 800 mg/serving). Their serving size is so small, however, that most healthy adults would eat several servings. Even some of the packaged soups that appear to be so healthy contain hundreds of milligrams of sodium per container (ramen noodles, for example).

On the plus side, sodium is an essential electrolyte, balanced with potassium. Sodium is used to produce cellular electricity, and the "spark" between these two minerals drive nerve transmissions along the axon and dendrite.

High-sodium packaged meals contain little to no potassium, so the electrical system of the body is put into jeopardy. Remember also that the rhythm of the heart is driven by electricity generated between the electrolytes. It is very important that the natural balance between sodium and potassium is maintained, not only for the health of the heart, but for the rest of the body.

One of the symptoms of too much sodium and too little potassium (found in dark green leafy vegetables) is exhaustion. Could this be one of the reasons American women are always tired?

A natural diet provides lots of potassium and essential amounts of sodium. The salt shaker is not needed to provide sodium! Some processed foods contain more than eight different forms of sodium. Eating these foods places a huge burden on the kidneys and adrenal glands, which must eliminate the excess sodium and try to maintain appropriate potassium levels. If the adrenal glands are already burdened by stress, excessive sodium consumption places another load on these organs. They simply may not be able to keep up—possibly stimulating heart arrhythmias, lack of energy production, and other symptoms.

Sugar

Sugar is a powerful lure. Humans ate an average of 10 pounds of sugar per year two-hundred years ago, points out nutritionist Ann-Louise Gittleman, author of *Get the Sugar Out* (Crown Publishing Group, 1996). Today, however, we are eating an average of 152 pounds of sugar per year, in addition to artificial sweeteners. Government studies show that the average American eats more than two hundred pounds of both sugar and artificial sweeteners per year.

Although diet has changed dramatically, the human body has changed very little. Gittleman writes,

> Our bodies simply haven't had time to respond and adapt to this nutrient-poor source of calories—and it appears that our bodies are rebelling with a multitude of physical complaints, telling us loudly and clearly that they don't like what they're being fed.[21]

Reduced levels of HDL cholesterol are associated with high sugar intake. Sugar sabotages the heart in other ways, too. First, it contributes to weight gain, which is implicated in heart disease. Second, it can throw blood sugar levels out of balance. If you have diabetes, excessive sugar intake increases the risk of complications such as heart disease.

While many experts loudly assert, "sugar has no effect on the brain or the rest of the body," other experts protest just as vehemently. Several years ago, researcher Dr. Gerald Reaven began studying a curious set of symptoms that, in a cluster, increased the risk of heart disease. The symptoms included high triglycerides, high cholesterol (particularly high LDL cholesterol), and abdominal or upper-body obesity or excess weight. Dr. Reaven found that the common factor in this cluster of symptoms was elevated circulating insulin.

He named this condition Syndrome X. The condition is characterized by insulin resistance. When insulin is secreted by the pancreas in response to elevated blood sugar, the hormone tries to "dock" onto the insulin receptor site on the cell wall. However, the receptor site becomes insensitive to the message of the hormone due to the continued intake of sugar and high–glycemic-index foods (bread, pasta, potatoes, white rice). Insulin is left circulating in the bloodstream. Because insulin's message was not received, blood sugar levels remain elevated, stimulating the pancreas to release even more insulin and sending insulin levels even higher.

Insulin resistance is also called carbohydrate sensitivity. These individuals are very sensitive to even small amounts of sugar. Yet they often continue to consume large amounts, completely oblivious to the damage taking place in their arteries and heart tissue.

SUGAR WOES

Refined sugar is present in soft drinks, packaged foods, table sugar, jams, syrups, baked goods, ice cream, breakfast cereals, and candy. It is also found in unlikely places: ketchup, nondairy creamer, frozen pizza, and salad dressing.

In addition, sugary foods may replace low-calorie, high-nutrient treats such as fruit. Sugar, including the fructose in fruits, should not make up more than 10 percent of our daily calorie intake.

A study of postmenopausal women illustrated Reaven's findings. The study was small, with only ten healthy postmenopausal women. They were provided with two types of diets. The first one, the 60 percent carbohydrate diet, offered 15 percent protein, 60 percent carbohydrate, and 25 percent fat. The second one, the 40 percent carbohydrate diet, offered 15 percent protein, 40 percent carbohydrate, and 45 percent fat.

Researchers found that levels of fasting triglycerides, VLDL triglycerides, and VLDL cholesterol were higher, and that HDL cholesterol levels were lower in the subjects on the 60 percent carbohydrate diet. From 8 A.M. to noon, plasma insulin and triglyceride levels were also higher with the 60 percent carbohydrate diet versus the 40 percent carbohydrate diet.

The study found that postmeal, the concentrations of insulin and triglyceride-rich lipoproteins were higher when sugar replaced fat in the diet. (This is a major flaw in the "low-fat craze" in the food industry.) LDL cholesterol concentrations were similar in both diets.

Researchers concluded that the more insulin resistant the individual became, the more likely that the low-fat, high-carbohydrate diet (the typical American reducing diet) would produce ischemic heart disease.[22]

Cholesterol

Dietary cholesterol is beneficial to the body, in reasonable amounts. This soft, waxy substance is an essential part of all cell membranes. It is present in the heart, nervous system, liver, skin, and muscle. Cholesterol generates bile acids, vitamin D, sex hormones, and adrenal hormones. The adrenal hormones control water and electrolyte balance, and the metabolism of fats, proteins, and carbohydrates.

Is cholesterol a "good guy" or a "bad guy"? Does dietary cholesterol increase the risk of heart disease, or is it an essential nutrient? It all depends.

Your liver produces most of the cholesterol you need. In fact, it produces the same amount of cholesterol that is found in eighty-eight pats of butter every day, regardless of dietary intake. In fact, when cholesterol intake is reduced, the liver may produce even more of it to meet the structural and functional demands of the body.

The problem is that Americans often consume too much cholesterol and saturated fat, particularly in the absence of other types of beneficial oils and antioxidant nutrients in the form of fresh fruits and vegetables. In other words, it is not necessary to eliminate all dietary cholesterol; we simply have to learn to eat a more balanced diet. Along with saturated fat and trans-fatty acids, dietary cholesterol can raise total cholesterol levels. High cholesterol levels are implicated in atherosclerosis, strokes, and heart disease. However, just reducing dietary cholesterol may do little to reduce serum cholesterol.

WHERE IS IT?

Dietary cholesterol is present in eggs, cheese, butter, lard, pork, beef, and shellfish. Plant foods do not contain cholesterol. Liver and other organ meats are low in fat but high in cholesterol.

So, What's for Dinner?

Putting all this information into a format that makes it easy for a woman to prepare a meal should not be difficult. Let's put the science aside. Let's stop listening to the experts as they argue among themselves. Let's stop worrying about the details and the conflicting information.

We simply have to get back to eating real food, as close to nature as possible, as fresh as possible, and as balanced as possible.

What Is a "Real Food Diet"?

Before the turn of the twentieth century, doctors treated very little heart disease because people were still, for the most part, eating real food. Because transportation was slow and refrigeration primitive, people tended to eat close to home, with farm-raised fruits and vegetables and wild animals raised on their natural foods. People ate seasonally and locally. They ate organic. They ate tree-ripened fruits and the vegetables they plucked out of the garden. About the only processing they did was to store the vegetables in the root cellar for the winter or to can the produce raised in their home gardens.

When one tries to make sense of epidemiological data, one begins to understand that food traditions around the world vary greatly. Some cultures eat few animal products; other cultures live almost totally on animal products. Some cultures eat few grains; other cultures eat a great deal of whole grains. Some cultures totally avoid dairy products other than mother's own milk; other cultures worship cream fresh from the cow's udder.

Some of these cultures enjoy vibrant health and live to ripe old ages (unless they die prematurely from poor sanitation, diseases introduced from the outside world, or accidents). What is the common thread that runs through these healthier cultures? They eat real food, grown in their part of the world. In other words, they eat locally, organically, seasonally, and fresh. How does this translate into our American food culture?

Here are some simple rules to follow when planning family meals that can protect and heal the heart:

1. Enjoy a wide variety of fresh fruits and vegetables selected from the fresh produce section of your supermarket or, even better, from local farmers' markets. If possible, eat organic, tree-ripened fruit and vegetables that are fresh and seasonal.

2. Enjoy one or two servings of legumes each day, to get plenty of good fiber and key minerals.

3. Enjoy an appropriate amount of protein foods daily, preferably divided into three meals. The average woman requires from 45 to 65 grams of protein per day. The average man requires from 55 to 75 grams per day. Some people require a little more protein; learn to listen to your body. If you are selecting vegetarian sources of protein, be sure to include adequate amounts of essential amino acids such as methionine and cysteine. These are necessary for the liver's detoxification pathways. Also, try to avoid eating the same type of protein food each day, as repeated consumption can increase the likelihood of developing food allergies to the protein. You must also make sure that your diet is adequate in zinc, vitamin B_{12}, folic acid, and essential fatty acids.

4. Enjoy an appropriate amount of fats each day, especially olive oil, flaxseed oil, and small amounts of butter. Avoid margarine and other hydrogenated oils.

5. Drink lots of fresh, pure water! Many nutritionists and nutritionally trained physicians recommend drinking 1 ounce of water for every 2 pounds of body weight. For example, a 150-pound person should drink 75 ounces of water per day. Water is needed to hydrate the body, cleanse the tissues, activate hundreds of thousands of enzymes, and perform many other functions in your system. Water is your best choice; other beverages do not adequately hydrate the body.

6. Include supplementary fiber such as psyllium and a blend of natural fiber. Fiber is needed to keep the colon functioning properly, to keep excess cholesterol swept out of the large intestine, to prevent

the reabsorption of used estrogens, and for many other functions. Up to 65 grams of fiber daily is recommended for the health of the colon and heart.

If you follow these simple guidelines, avoid processed foods, and eat like a cavewoman, chances are that you'll greatly reduce your risk of developing heart disease. You may even heal your heart, if damage has already occurred.

CHAPTER 6

Making Up for the Standard American Diet

When you look at what Americans eat, it is obvious that trying to heal the heart in the context of our food culture is a lost cause. In fact, the American food culture appears to be a key contributing factor in heart disease.

Women are in trouble dietwise for a number of reasons. We have become increasingly dependent on processed foods. Few of us are old enough to remember when food was really food. Most of us grew up on Betty Crocker, McDonald's, Spam, and infant formula. We drink dozens of gallons of soft drinks, coffee, tea, and alcoholic beverages. We drink very little water.

We eat fewer than two servings of fruits and vegetables per day and a quarter of those servings are in the form of French fries. We eat more reconstituted potatoes than real potatoes, more strawberry ice cream than fresh strawberries, and—well, the bad news just keeps getting worse. Do you want to visually understand what people eat? Just stroll through your local supermarket and take note of the products lining the shelves. Notice how small the fresh produce section is, compared with the frozen food section or the snack food section. Notice how little area is devoted to fresh seafood or organic chicken, and you'll see why we are in deep trouble nutritionally.

American women are struggling with long-term malnutrition due to the diet industry. Well over 50 percent of American women are overweight, and most are on some type of weight loss diet. Virtually all of those diet plans fail, but that does not deter them. They'll buy the next best-seller diet book on the market and try that one, too, only to fail again.

Virtually every diet program on the market today is based on malnutrition of some sort. Low-fat diets create deficiencies in essential fatty acids, fats that are very important to the health of the heart and the entire body. High-protein diets can create problems for the heart, kidneys, liver, and bones, and are seriously deficient in heart-essential nutrients such as magnesium and zinc. Low-calorie diets may lead to a calorie deficit, as well as deficiencies in B-complex vitamins, zinc, iron, vitamin C, essential fatty acids, and other nutrients. High-carbohydrate diets undersupply protein and fat, as well as several minerals and other nutrients. They set dieters up for the development of Syndrome X and diabetes.

If you have been on a diet, your body may still be struggling to maintain health. If you have repeatedly dieted over the years, you may be starving to death. To heal your heart, you will have to pay close attention to both diet and supplementation.

Maximizing the diet is critically important; we have already established that. But given the fact that we must compensate for years of malnutrition, we need to take a serious look at supplements that can *supplement* the diet. Notice the emphasis on the word *supplement*. A dietary supplement, as important as it is, will never *supplant* real food. We must add the supplement to a healthy diet. Decades of solid research has firmly established the benefits of adding specific nutrients to a balanced diet to help prevent heart disease and/or stop its progression.

The first recommendation is that every woman should be taking a well-balanced vitamin and mineral supplement that provides, at the very minimum, a base amount of every essential nutrient. Most supplements undersupply essential minerals such as calcium, magnesium, and zinc. Minerals take up a great deal of space in a capsule or tablet, and to get the heart-protective dosage of minerals, one should expect to take several capsules per day. It is impossible to find a high-quality, one-a-day tablet.

Interestingly, one colonic expert noted that she frequently saw intact vitamin supplements floating through the colonic machinery, with the writing still readable. Apparently the hard, compressed tablets didn't break down in the environment of the stomach!

Beyond the daily vitamin/mineral formula, it will frequently be necessary to include additional nutrients to your supplement program, just for added insurance. In the sections that follow, we will discuss some of the specific nutrients needed to heal the heart.

Folic Acid and Vitamins B$_6$ and B$_{12}$

Although serum cholesterol has received the biggest press splash over the past few years, another marker may be even more important than cholesterol levels in predicting a heart event or protecting a healthy heart. That marker is a little-known protein called homocysteine.

Homocysteine is a metabolic by-product of the metabolism of methionine, an essential amino acid. Homocysteine is naturally present in the human body. However, the medical community now recognizes that when homocysteine levels begin to soar above normal physiological levels, one's risk for heart and blood vessel damage increases dramatically. High homocysteine may also be implicated in Alzheimer's disease.[1]

Harvard-trained researcher Kilmer S. McCully, M.D., pioneered the research into homocysteine's role in heart disease over the past forty years. His research shows that the incidence of heart disease in the United States is directly linked to high homocysteine levels. Excess homocysteine is associated with the typical low-nutrient, high-calorie standard American diet, which includes too many processed and refined foods and too few fresh, natural foods. When foods are processed, the B-complex vitamins are essentially stripped out, leaving a critical deficiency in three vitamins needed to keep homocysteine levels within normal biological ranges: vitamin B$_6$, vitamin B$_{12}$, and folic acid. It is the shortage of these three nutrients that leads to a buildup of homocysteine.

Researchers discovered the connection between vitamin B deficiencies and homocysteine levels by studying a genetic disease called *homocystinuria*. Vitamin B$_6$, vitamin B$_{12}$, and folic acid are cofactors for three enzymes that metabolize homocysteine through the normal metabolic channels, and when these nutrients are absent or deficient (as in the standard American diet, for example), homocysteine levels rise, causing an increased risk of heart disease.

At this point, the evidence suggests that lowering high homocysteine levels by optimizing B-complex intake may decrease the risk of cardiovascular disease.

The recommended amount is very modest: 400 mcg of folic acid, 3 mg of vitamin B$_6$, and 15 mcg of vitamin B$_{12}$ daily. Most multivitamin/mineral formulas contain these nutrients in the right amounts.

Since vitamin B_6, vitamin B_{12}, and folic acid may normalize homocysteine levels, it is a good idea to get enough of these nutrients. Fortunately, it is not difficult to ensure this level of nutrition in a well-balanced diet. Vitamin B_6 is plentiful in poultry, fish, pork, eggs, soybeans, oats, peanuts, and bananas. Vitamin B_{12} is available in meat, fish, poultry, dairy products, nutritional yeast, fortified soymilk, soy products, and some cereals. Folic acid is found in liver, leafy vegetables, and citrus foods. Furthermore, the Food and Drug Administration (FDA) now requires that breads, cereal, pasta, and other grain-based foods be fortified with folic acid.

Because it is easy to perform and inexpensive, many physicians recommend getting a homocysteine test done to ensure your level is not too high.

Niacin

Niacin, also known as vitamin B_3, is a popular natural remedy for balancing cholesterol levels. Specifically, it appears to increase HDL cholesterol and stimulate circulation. Some studies have also shown niacin to reduce triglycerides and total cholesterol, particularly in individuals with diabetes. It may also reduce lipoprotein (a), another marker for heart disease.[2]

One study compared niacin with atorvastatin, a widely used lipid-lowering drug. The researchers concluded that while atorvastatin appeared to lower LDL cholesterol levels, niacin also had a favorable effect on HDL levels.[3] In other words, niacin not only helped lower total cholesterol, but helped improve the HDL/LDL levels of the cholesterol fraction.

Michael T. Murray, N.D., reports that inositol hexaniacinate is the preferred form of niacin. This form has been used in Europe for decades to lower total cholesterol. Not only does inositol hexaniacinate deliver better results than standard niacin, Dr. Murray says, but it is better tolerated in the human system. Inositol hexaniacinate also promotes healthy blood flow. Because of this, it has been successfully used in alleviating painful muscle cramps (intermittent claudication) due to limited blood flow.

How Much Niacin Is Recommended?

Pellagra is a niacin-deficiency disease characterized by lesions of the skin and mouth and gastrointestinal symptoms. While this condition is rare in the

United States today, niacin deficiency is not as rare. Other signs of niacin deficiency include irritability, insomnia, fatigue, indigestion, and recurring headaches.

The recommended dietary allowance (RDA) for niacin: for females aged eleven to fifty, 15 mg; for women fifty-one and older, 13 mg; for pregnant women, 17 mg; and for lactating women, 20 mg.

Niacin can be toxic in high doses. Amounts over 2 grams may contribute to skin discoloration and dryness, reduced glucose tolerance, high uric-acid levels, and aggravation of peptic ulcers. Excess niacin can also lead to liver damage, particularly when using the time-release form of the vitamin. Megadoses of niacin are not recommended without close medical supervision— liver damage may result.

High doses of nicotinic acid—the form of niacin commonly used to lower cholesterol levels—can lead to the infamous "niacin flush," characterized by tingling, intense flushing, and throbbing in the head caused by dilation of the blood vessels that lie close to the skin. These symptoms last only about fifteen minutes, and although they're uncomfortable, they're not dangerous.

Niacinamide, a derivative of niacin, does not have these side effects; however, it does not affect cholesterol or triglyceride levels.

Foods rich in niacin include dried brewer's yeast, wheat bran, nuts, pig liver, chicken, soy flour, fatty fish, wheat grains, cheese, dried fruits, brown rice, wheat germ, oat flakes, eggs, and legumes.

Vitamin C

Vitamin C may be one of the most visible heroes of the natural health movement, thanks, in part, to the outstanding work of Linus Pauling, Ph.D. He studied this important nutrient for decades and published many works on the results of his research.

Pauling and other researchers found that animals left in their natural, wild environment produce many grams of vitamin C per day. In contrast, humans are one of the few "animals" who are unable to manufacture their own vitamin C; we lack a crucial enzyme needed to convert carbohydrates into vitamin C. We must depend on food sources to provide this valuable antiaging, health-protective nutrient. Unfortunately, however, most Americans do not consume even close to the amount of vitamin C that Pauling and his associates have found to be truly heart (and health) protective.

Dr. Pauling and associates found that high levels of heart-damaging lipoprotein (a) are associated with low levels of ascorbic acid (vitamin C).[4] Conversely, a high intake of vitamin C is associated with lower levels of LDL cholesterol and higher levels of HDL cholesterol.

One study, involving ten patients with coronary heart failure, explored the impact of vitamin C on CHF. The researchers found that it helped thin the blood and improve endothelial function, "suggesting a potential role for vitamin C as a therapeutic agent in CHF."[5]

How Much Vitamin C Is Recommended?

As an antioxidant, vitamin C protects against the free radical damage associated with atherosclerosis, as well as cancer, cataracts, and other age-related conditions.

Humans cannot produce or store their own vitamin C. Because vitamin C is a water-soluble nutrient, the body quickly rids itself of any excess. Therefore, humans need fresh supplies of vitamin C by way of fruits, vegetables, and supplements. That's what makes vitamin C, also known as ascorbic acid, an "essential" nutrient.

Scurvy is the classic disease of vitamin C deficiency. Although this condition was much more widespread in the nineteenth century, it still occasionally occurs today, particularly in mild forms. Symptoms of scurvy include muscle weakness, bleeding or swollen gums, loss of teeth, impaired wound healing, fatigue, and depression. Some clinicians believe that heart disease itself is a symptom of vitamin C deficiency.

The body uses up vitamin C very quickly, so there is virtually no risk of toxic accumulation. If you take more than 1,000 mg daily, you may start to urinate more often or experience mild diarrhea.

Some research suggests that as little as 500 mg daily of ascorbic acid may exert a pro-oxidant effect, and thereby damage healthy cells. Vitamin C increases iron absorption, so individuals with certain blood disorders (hemochromatosis, thalassemia, or sideroblastic anemia) should limit their intake. However, one review suggests that although vitamin C may have a pro-oxidant effect in the presence of transition metals such as iron or copper, it has not been found to otherwise increase the oxidative damage in the living organism.[6]

Dietary sources of vitamin C include oranges, lemons, limes, tangerines, grapefruits, rose hips, acerola cherries, papayas, cantaloupes, and strawberries. Vegetables rich in vitamin C include red and green peppers, broccoli, Brussels sprouts, tomatoes, asparagus, parsley, dark leafy greens, and cabbage. Natural ascorbic acid supplements typically include rose hips, acerola cherries, peppers, or citrus fruits.

Vitamin E

Vitamin E is another incredibly important nutrient, especially known for its work in protecting the heart. This complex of vitamins (tocopherols) has been studied for decades, and overwhelming evidence indicates that high levels of vitamin E protect the heart and the entire cardiovascular system. This fat-soluble nutrient is best known for its antioxidant function, protecting the cells' tissues, and fat throughout the body, from oxidation. It also helps thin the blood, thereby reducing the risk of dangerous blood clots.

One study focused on 5,133 Finnish women and men who were free of heart disease at the beginning of the study. After fourteen years, 244 participants had died of coronary heart disease. Researchers found a significant inverse correlation between vitamin E intake and heart disease deaths in both women and men. The women who ingested the most vitamin E faced a 65 percent lower risk of heart disease than the women who took the least.[7]

How Much Vitamin E Is Recommended?

Severe vitamin E deficiencies are uncommon. If you are cutting fatty foods out of your diet, though, you may not be getting enough vitamin E. Particularly at risk are the elderly, the sick, people who take certain medications, or anyone who smokes, drinks alcohol, and/or is exposed to excessive radiation from the sun. In addition, food processing, refining, and storage deplete the vitamin E content of many foods.

There are no clear-cut symptoms of vitamin E deficiency. However, deficits of this nutrient can impair your antioxidant defenses.

The RDA for women aged eighteen and older is 24 IU. However, 400 to 800 mg daily is recommended for optimal antioxidant protection.

Although vitamin E is a fat-soluble nutrient, as much as 800 IU is considered safe. However, supplemental vitamin E is not recommended for individuals with blood-coagulation problems or who take anticoagulants. In fact, if you are planning to have surgery, do not take supplemental vitamin E for two weeks before and after surgery, and tell your doctor if you have been taking vitamin E supplements.

With all the vitamin products available, choosing the best vitamin E supplement can be confusing. Natural vitamin E (d-alpha-tocopherol) is a better choice than synthetic vitamin E (dl-alpha-tocopherol). A landmark laboratory study found that natural vitamin E remained in the tissues much longer than its synthetic counterpart.[8]

Coenzyme Q10 (CoQ10)

Because CoQ10 is such a remarkable nutrient for the cardiovascular system, we will discuss it in greater detail in Chapter 7. Here we will give you the short version.

CoQ10 is also known as ubiquinone or ubiquinol. Ubiquinone (as in ubiquitous) refers to CoQ10's presence in every plant and animal cell. CoQ10 is a potent antioxidant nutrient that is naturally present in all the tissues of the body.

Human cells contain small enclosures called mitochondria. These mitochondria generate energy by breaking down sugars, fats, and amino acids. CoQ10 exists in the cells' mitochondria and is an integral part of the body's production of energy.

CoQ10 has been used to treat individuals with congestive heart failure.[9] This supplement may be added to, or used to replace, digitalis, diuretics, or other drugs designed to improve the pumping of the heart. However, close medical supervision is essential.

"In patients with chronic heart failure, the addition of CoQ10 to conventional therapy reduces the hospitalization rate for worsening of heart failure and the incidence of serious cardiovascular complications," writes Dr. C. Morisco from the University of Degli Studi Federico II, Napoli, Italy. Morisco and his colleagues conducted a double-blind, placebo-controlled study on CoQ10 and heart health. They found that this supplement significantly improved the amount of blood pumped by the heart.[10]

In addition, CoQ10 protects LDL and HDL lipoproteins from oxidation, or free-radical damage.[11] It also appears to lower high blood pressure.[12]

How Much CoQ10 Is Recommended?

So far, little has been published about CoQ10 deficiency. CoQ10 deficiency is a suspected factor in many cases of heart disease and chronic fatigue syndrome, however. Perhaps by addressing this deficiency, patients may take more control of their illnesses.

No recommended dietary allowance has been established for CoQ10. Physician and health writer Ray Sahelian, M.D., author of *Coenzyme Q10: Nature's Heart Energizer* (Impakt, 1997), recommends starting with a low dose of 10 mg daily. Those with heart disease may want to take 300 mg or more. Consult a health care professional, though, before taking high doses of CoQ10. Most people get 2 to 20 mg of CoQ10 daily through their diets.[13] Excessive doses of CoQ10 may lead to nausea, overstimulation, and insomnia. However, long-term use of CoQ10, in appropriate amounts, appears to be safe.[14]

There is scant research on the combination of CoQ10 with heart medications such as diuretics, antiarrhythmic agents, blood pressure medicines, and digitalis. Always consult your physician before combining medicines, natural or otherwise.

Vitamin E and CoQ10 work well together to prevent free radical damage in the body.[15] CoQ10 is found in fish and meat, and it is also available as a supplement.

Carotenoids

Carotenoids may be another unsung nutritional hero. Almost every study examining the impact of good nutrition on the heart shows a benefit to eating foods that are rich in this important family of nutrients. The advice to "eat our colors," is not just a clever statement. It is an important concept because colorful foods are rich in carotenoids. Besides their antioxidant value, carotenoid-containing foods are high in fiber, another benefit to the heart.

Carotenoids are naturally occurring pigments in plants and are responsible for the bright colors of fruits and vegetables, especially dark green, leafy vegetables. These nutrients convert to vitamin A in the liver, as needed. Bioflavonoids (carotenoids) apparently perform their own biological function as well, apart from merely converting into the fat-soluble vitamin A.

More than five hundred different carotenoids have been identified. These include alpha-carotene, beta-carotene, lycopene, zeaxanthin, lutein, and astaxanthin. Few of these powerful nutrients have been studied in depth to discover their benefits to the body. As scientists have examined a few of these bioflavonoids, however, some common benefits seem to emerge. Bioflavonoids are powerful antioxidants; they protect the body against free radical mischief that not only damages the heart tissue but contributes to premature aging in every part of the body.

Because they are potent antioxidants, carotenoids appear to reduce the risk of heart disease. One study examined the association between diet and atherosclerosis in more than 12,000 women and men. Researchers found that participants who consumed diets highest in carotenoids had the lowest incidence of atherosclerosis.[16]

What Level of Carotenoids Is Recommended?

Symptoms of vitamin A deficiency include night blindness; skin problems, such as thickened, dry skin and keratin (hardened bumps of protein); cirrhosis of the liver; and susceptibility to infection.

A daily dose of 25,000 IU, or 15 mg of beta-carotene, has been recommended. Specific recommendations are not available for the hundreds of other carotenoids. However, a diet rich in fruits and vegetables is believed to supply sufficient levels of these nutrients.

Although vitamin A can be toxic at high doses, carotenoids are considered safe. Certain individuals who take large amounts of beta-carotene report loose stools, but this usually clears up on its own. Consuming high amounts of carotenoid-rich foods or supplements, for a prolonged period of time, can cause the skin to turn orange in certain people. Fortunately, this effect is not dangerous, and it is reversible.

A deficiency of zinc, vitamin C, protein, or thyroid hormone can sabotage the conversion of carotenoids to vitamin A.

Fruits and vegetables are the richest dietary sources of carotenoids. Apricots, cantaloupe, carrots, green, leafy vegetables, pumpkin, sweet potato, and winter squash provide a wealth of beta-carotene. Carrots and pumpkins also contain alpha-carotene. Lutein and zeaxanthin are available in green, leafy vegetables, pumpkin, and red pepper. Guava, pink grapefruit, tomatoes and tomato products, and watermelon all supply lycopene. Cryptoxanthin is found in mangoes, nectarines, oranges, papaya, peaches, and tangerines.

Even though a great deal of emphasis has been placed on improving our dietary status, Americans seem to avoid fresh fruits and vegetables, rich sources of carotenoids. We're going backwards in the vegetable department. Carotenoid intake may actually be *decreasing* in the United States.

What happens to your body when you're not getting enough carotenoids? A one-hundred-day study explored the effect of a low-carotenoid diet on nine premenopausal women. Researchers found that carotenoids helped prevent lipid peroxidation in the cells.[17] Lipid peroxidation is implicated in atherosclerosis and heart disease.

L-Carnitine

L-carnitine, an amino acid, is the active form of carnitine. It is produced in the liver and kidneys and stored in the heart and skeletal muscle. It is also concentrated in the brain and in sperm. Like water-soluble vitamins, L-carnitine appears to be easily and completely absorbed by the body.

Among its other uses, L-carnitine may improve heart function in individuals with congestive heart failure.[18] In fact, L-carnitine supplementation is highly recommended for individuals with heart disease. Author Michael T. Murray, N.D., explains that if the heart is not getting enough oxygen, L-carnitine levels in the body quickly decrease. L-carnitine supplements can help stabilize the carnitine levels in the heart, thereby helping the heart muscle use its limited oxygen supply more efficiently.[19]

According to an animal study, L-carnitine appears to support cardiovascular health by raising HDL cholesterol and lowering LDL cholesterol (Diaz, 2000).[20] While L-carnitine is moving fats from your bloodstream into your cells, it is keeping these fats from forming plaque on your arteries.

L-carnitine also benefits the heart through indirect mechanisms:

1. It helps reduce insulin resistance, an important contributing factor to both diabetes and heart disease.[21]

2. It appears to increase exercise tolerance in individuals with chronic stable angina.[22]
3. Because of its fat-burning properties, L-carnitine helps control weight. Obesity is a major contributing factor in heart disease.

How Much L-Carnitine Is Recommended?

Although a healthy body usually synthesizes enough L-carnitine for its needs, there are certain populations for whom this may be an essential supplement. Without sufficient levels of L-carnitine, the body does not burn fats normally, thereby leading to impaired protein and carbohydrate metabolism.

One serious by-product of L-carnitine deficiency is elevated fats in the blood. This buildup of fats eventually forms plaque on the arteries.

Carnitine is derived from the Latin word *carnis*, which means red meat. Red meat is the richest dietary source of L-carnitine. In general, the redder the meat, the more carnitine it has. Smaller amounts are found in fish, poultry, milk products, and fermented soybeans. If you are concerned about the high content of saturated fat, hormones, and antibiotics found in most red meat, take supplemental L-carnitine instead.

Use L-carnitine, not D-carnitine. D-carnitine is the inactive form of carnitine and may dilute the benefit of L-carnitine. In one study, a mixture of D- and L-carnitine made it much more difficult for patients with angina to exercise.[23]

On the other hand, L-carnitine appears to work synergistically with both coenzyme Q10 and pantethine, a derivative of pantothenic acid. Also, choline may help conserve carnitine, and increase carnitine levels in the cells.[24]

The recommended daily amount of L-carnitine is 1,500 to 4,000 mg in divided doses.[25]

Potassium

Minerals do not work in isolation in the human body. They are frequently paired with other minerals that have opposing functions, or otherwise balance the effects of these powerful ionic tools. For example, calcium needs to be balanced with magnesium to maintain a steady nerve pulse. Zinc is an oppositional mineral with copper; when these two essential nutrients get out of balance, serious mental and physical symptoms can emerge. Potassium's "marital partner" is sodium; both are electrolytes that provide the electrical current of the nervous system and help provide for the production of cellular energy.

We do not have any trouble getting enough sodium in this country; in fact, we get far too much sodium as our love affair with processed foods grows. Pick up any package or container of processed foods, even "healthy" frozen entrees. You will see huge amounts of sodium without its companion mineral, potassium.

We know that excessive salt consumption can lead to elevated blood pressure and water retention, both of which are dangerous to the heart. We know that an imbalance of sodium and potassium leads to energy loss and irritability. We also know that this imbalance is easily corrected: simply add more fresh fruits and vegetables to the diet. Vegetables are rich in potassium, with small (physiologically balanced) amounts of sodium.

How Much Potassium Is Recommended?

If you have hypertension, your health care provider may recommend supplemental potassium. Among other benefits, potassium helps to lower blood pressure and reduce your risk of stroke. As people consume more potassium, they excrete sodium, which helps keep blood pressure in balance.

Key electrolytes in your system include potassium, sodium, chloride, calcium, magnesium, and water. Healthy functioning of your cardiovascular system, brain, nerves, and muscles depends on the proper ratio of electrolytes. For optimal wellness, the body needs to carefully regulate these electrolytes within very narrow limits. It does this by transporting them into or out of the cells.

If you are not getting enough potassium, your electrolytes can be thrown out of balance. An electrolyte imbalance can lead to faulty heart rhythm, as well as spasms, impaired athletic ability and strength, and even sudden death.

Unfortunately, shortages of potassium are not uncommon. The standard American diet emphasizes processed and convenience foods, often high in sodium and fat. It does not include an abundance of fruits, vegetables, and other plant foods. Yet plant foods are the richest sources of potassium.

Furthermore, a salt-rich diet can significantly deplete your body's stores of potassium. If you eat a lot of salt, you may need to increase your potassium intake. Magnesium deficiency may also lead to potassium deficiency.

You should be getting 1,600 to 5,625 mg of potassium daily. Symptoms of potassium deficiency include weakness, loss of appetite, nausea, listlessness, irrational behavior, muscle weakness, and irregular heartbeat.

Too much potassium can also pose health risks. Some potassium-sparing diuretics and ACE inhibitors can lead to potassium accumulation. If you take these types of blood pressure medications, avoid potassium supplements or salt substitutes that contain potassium. Generally, you can maintain safe potassium levels by eating unprocessed plant foods.

Moreover, people with heart disease or kidney disease should not take potassium supplements without consulting their physicians. With kidney disease, the concern is that potassium can build up to potentially toxic levels, because the kidneys are unable to maintain the proper balance. However, one study involving six adult dialysis patients indicated that high potassium intake may not be such a threat after all. For three months, the patients used a dialysate (the material that passes through the membrane in dialysis) that contained no potassium. Over the following three months, they used a dialysate that did contain potassium. Researchers found that total body potassium concentrations remained the same.[26] More research is needed in this area.

The following foods are especially rich in potassium: apples, avocados, bananas, beets, blackberries, cantaloupe, cherries, cooked spinach, grapefruit, green lima beans, honeydew melon, lentils, milk, orange juice, potatoes with skin, prunes, raisins, red beans, strawberries, tomato juice, and watermelon. Potassium is also available as a supplement.

Calcium

When we think of calcium, we think of bones, and rightly so. By far, the greatest deposit of calcium in the human body is in the hard structure of the bones, where it provides the rigidity needed for the body's skeletal framework.

But calcium is also used for other bodily functions. For example, it stimulates the nerve cells to contract, and in opposition to magnesium, helps regulate the heartbeat and muscle tone of other muscles. If the delicate calcium/magnesium balance is thrown into disarray by the overconsumption of calcium and the underconsumption of magnesium, muscles become rigid and taut, and the heart rate is seriously dysregulated.

Calcium supports healthy heart rhythm and helps lower blood pressure by relaxing the blood vessels in individuals with essential hypertension.[27]

Specifically, calcium may help prevent the development of pregnancy-induced hypertension and preeclampsia, a serious condition associated with elevations in blood pressure, fluid retention, and loss of protein in the urine.

How Much Calcium Is Recommended?

Fully 50 percent of American women do not get the recommended dietary allowance (RDA) for calcium. Low calcium intake contributes to high blood pressure, as well as to osteoporosis, colon cancer, premenstrual syndrome, and rickets.

Excessive amounts of magnesium, zinc, fiber, and oxalates negatively affect calcium absorption. In addition, tobacco use, caffeine, alcohol, carbonated soft drinks, phosphates, protein, sodium, and sugar increase calcium excretion. Aluminum-containing antacids ultimately lead to an increase in bone breakdown and calcium excretion.

The RDA for females aged eleven to twenty-four is 1,200 mg; for females twenty-four years and older, 800 mg; and for pregnant or lactating females, 1,200 mg. However, the National Academy of Sciences recommends higher levels of calcium: 1,000 mg for adults nineteen to fifty years old, and 1,200 mg daily for adults aged fifty-one and older. Up to 2,000 mg of calcium daily is considered very safe.

Some researchers express concern that increased calcium intake may lead to calcium oxalate kidney stones. Calcium citrate appears to bypass this justifiable concern. Although urinary calcium rises in individuals consuming calcium citrate, this form of calcium appears to inhibit the formation of kidney stones.

Paradoxically, *low* calcium intake may contribute to the development of kidney stones. In one study, the researchers concluded, "We believe that an adequate dose of calcium can normalize urinary oxalate excretion."[28]

Foods rich in calcium include black beans, brick cheese, broccoli, canned salmon, collard greens, dried pinto beans, garbanzo beans, hazelnuts, hulled sesame seeds, kale, kelp, milk, mustard greens, parsley, sardines, spinach, sunflower seeds, tofu, turnip greens, wheat and barley grass, and yogurt. Calcium formulas are also available.

Calcium can be difficult to absorb and utilize. Vitamin D is required for calcium absorption and placement into bone tissue.

Women may be lulled into complacency about their calcium levels because they consume a lot of dairy products. However, processed dairy foods (pasteurized, homogenized milk and cheese products) are poor sources of calcium. According to World Health Organization figures, up to 80 percent of the world's population may be intolerant to dairy products and as such, should avoid eating processed dairy foods. Milk and milk-based products are among the top three allergens, and many nutritionists recommend avoiding dairy products altogether.

If dairy is avoided, what then becomes of our calcium status? A discussion of osteoporosis is beyond the scope of this book. However, countries and cultures that do not consume dairy products past weaning, and who eat prodigious amounts of fresh and sea vegetables, suffer from osteoporosis far less than women in our culture who load up on cheese and ice cream and still believe the adage, "Milk does a body good." Bone protection is conferred by the balance of trace nutrients, the absence of coffee and soft-drink consumption, exercise, and other lifestyle factors that help lower the risk of bone disease.

Bones and heart tissue do not have competing interests. If we eat a diet that is good for the heart, it is good for the bones, too. The whole discussion of how much calcium protects against osteoporosis and heart disease is moot if we can just get back to our ancestral tradition. This entails eating copious amounts of fruits and vegetables, and *not* stuffing our bodies with soft drinks, sugar, and coffee.

Magnesium

Calcium is getting all the press, but it should be sharing the limelight with its companion mineral, magnesium. This mineral is closely linked with heart health (the entire cardiovascular system and the neurological system). More mainstream physicians are now recommending magnesium for patients with acute heart attacks, chronic cardiovascular disease, and heart arrhythmias.[29] This mineral also helps the muscles, including the heart muscle, work more effectively.[30] In addition, magnesium supplementation is highly recommended for people with diabetes, as magnesium deficiency is more pronounced in this population.

One study investigated the effects of magnesium deficiency on the rat common carotid artery. The researchers found significant alterations in the carotid arteries of magnesium-deficient rats. Specifically, they were stiffer. The authors of the study concluded, "Since magnesium deficiency is considered a risk factor, these mechanical alterations could contribute to the development of atherosclerosis, hypertension, and cardiovascular diseases."[31]

Patients suffering from myocardial infarction and congestive heart failure are frequently magnesium deficient. In patients with severe myocardial infarction, there was an increased incidence of ventricular ectopy with low magnesium levels.[32]

Magnesium deficiency is associated with cardiac arrhythmias, ischemic heart disease, hypertension,[33] congestive heart failure, premature ventricular contractions, ventricular tachycardia,[34] exercise-induced angina,[35] and increased susceptibility of lipoproteins to peroxidation (free radical damage).[36] Moreover, studies and clinical work have frequently shown that magnesium replacement after a heart attack improves the odds of recovery.[37]

Diets rich in calcium but poor in magnesium (lots of dairy products and not many dark green vegetables) are the problem. Calcium is a stimulating nutrient, exciting the nerve signal to activity, and triggering muscle contraction. On the other hand, magnesium is a relaxing mineral, causing the nerve signal to cease activity, and relaxing muscle contraction. When calcium is in proper balance with magnesium, the muscles (including the heart muscle) contract and relax . . . contract and relax . . . contract and relax . . . in a regular rhythm.

Overfeed the body with calcium and rob it of magnesium, and heart arrhythmias may well occur, sometimes to the point of a "heart event."

Magnesium is an incredibly versatile nutrient, involved in the metabolism of sugars, regulation of blood sugar, production of cellular energy, and activation of thousands of enzymes (many of which are brain and heart enzymes). So it stands to reason that a magnesium-poor diet will affect virtually every part of the body. The heart needs its share of magnesium and is often shortchanged in our green vegetable–deficient culture.

How Much Magnesium Is Recommended?

Magnesium deficiency has been implicated in cardiac arrhythmia, high blood pressure, and heart attack. Certain medications, such as diuretics, insulin, and digitalis, can reduce magnesium levels.

Factors contributing to magnesium deficiency include alcohol consumption, high intake of dietary fiber and phosphates (as in soft drinks), intense psychological stress, strenuous exercise, diuretic use, diarrhea, and high levels of zinc and vitamin D. In addition, high calcium intake, surgery, liver disease, kidney disease, and oral contraceptive use are associated with magnesium shortages.

The elderly are especially at risk for magnesium deficiency. Marginal magnesium deficits are also common among adolescents, dieters, those with diabetes, athletes, and women with osteoporosis. Symptoms of magnesium deficiency include rapid heartbeat, confusion, insomnia, irritability, poor digestion, muscle cramps, and seizures.

For adult women, the RDA for magnesium is 300 mg. Unfortunately, the standard American diet includes only 143 to 266 mg of magnesium daily; The human system requires more.

Magnesium overdose is rare. Signs of magnesium toxicity include nausea and vomiting, extreme muscle weakness, difficulty breathing, unusually low blood pressure, and irregular heartbeat. If you experience these symptoms, seek emergency medical treatment immediately.

In addition, magnesium supplements are not recommended for pregnant or lactating women, or people with kidney disease or severe heart disease, unless they are closely monitored by a qualified health care professional.

Magnesium is plentiful in seafood, especially bluefish, carp, cod, flounder, halibut, and herring. Other magnesium-rich foods include tofu, legumes, kelp, wheat bran, wheat germ, almonds, cashews, blackstrap molasses, brewer's yeast, Brazil nuts, and peanuts. Fruits and fruit juice, leafy green vegetables, sunflower seeds, and snails are also good dietary sources of magnesium. If you choose to take a magnesium supplement, choose a form that is readily absorbed, such as magnesium malate, succinate, fumarate, or citrate. The body has more difficulty using magnesium oxide, gluconate, sulfate, and chloride.

Also keep in mind that organic forms of magnesium are not as associated with diarrhea, while higher doses of inorganic magnesium salts can trigger this uncomfortable malady.

No nutrient is an island—magnesium included. Potassium depends on magnesium to help activate the sodium/potassium pump that pushes sodium out of, and potassium into, the cells. When magnesium is deficient, potassium is often lacking as well. This mineral works with calcium to promote

---

MAGNESIUM IS A NATURAL CALCIUM CHANNEL BLOCKER

When administered in combination with calcium channel blockers, magnesium may be used to treat hypertension. Magnesium works as a calcium channel blocker for several reasons, including blocking the entry of calcium via receptor-operated channels of vascular smooth muscle cells; within the cell, magnesium inhibits calcium release and drives it into the sarcoplasma reticulum, competes with calcium for binding sites in plasma membranes, and blocks the slow calcium channels. The net result is increased vessel dilation and reduced blood pressure.[22]

---

the strength of bones and teeth. Vitamin B_6 helps ensure that magnesium gets inside the cell.

Omega-3 Fatty Acids

In the United States in the late twentieth and early twenty-first centuries, fat has been a hard sell. For decades we have been told by the medical profession and mainstream press that fat is bad and harmful, and if we eat it, we'll die of a heart condition. We are "fat phobic."

Fat is, however, an essential nutrient, needed for literally every cell in the body. Fat is used to synthesize male and female hormones. It is embedded in the membrane of every body cell, contributing to the pliability of the cell membrane. This pliability means that nutrients can be carried into the cell environment, and toxic materials can be carried out of it. Saturated fats contribute to the rigidity of the cell membrane so that the cell retains its shape against the pressure of the surrounding cells.

Fats encase the myelin sheath, hastening the transmission of the nerve signal along the axon and the dendrite. Interruptions of the fatty tissue in the myelin sheath cause severe neurological disorders. In addition, fat is a preferred source of energy for the heart, especially after exercise or physical activity of long duration. Fat improves the texture of the skin, hair, and fingernails.

Low-fat diets are causally linked to fatigue, hypothyroidism, weight *gain*, hormone imbalance, depression, and other disorders. Clearly, promoters of low-fat diets are not working in our best interests, even in terms of heart health.

Again, keep in mind that a diet that is good for the heart is good for the rest of the body. If we adopt a particular type of diet to protect the cardiovascular system, we do not jeopardize the health of any other system.

As might be expected, all fats are not equal, although all fats were created equal. However, we've done enormous damage to dietary fats by processing the nutrition out of them and, in the end, creating harmful fats that damage the body.

So what are these fats that are so good for the body? Wholesome fats that improve cardiovascular health include the omega-3 fatty acids found in ocean-raised seafood, in flaxseed oil, and in smaller amounts of other vegetable sources of oils. Omega-6 fatty acids are also important to the body; however, we are consuming far too little of the omega-3 fats and far too much of the omega-6 fats. This throws off the natural balance between these essential nutrients.

Diets that are skewed in favor of omega-6 fatty acids may be proinflammatory and increase the risk of heart disease. Diets that favor omega-3 fatty acids are anti-inflammatory and confer protection to the heart and entire cardiovascular system. For good health, we need a balanced ratio of omega-3 and omega-6 essential fatty acids, somewhere in the range of 4:1. In other words, we should be getting four times more omega-3 than omega-6 fatty acids. Unfortunately, the typical North American diet supplies a disproportionate amount of omega-6 oils. Some data indicate that instead of a 4:1 ratio of omega-3 to omega-6, we are consuming a 20:1 omega-6 to omega-3. This dietary imbalance seriously jeopardizes the heart.

If low-fat, vegetarian diets are so good for the heart, why are the hearts of the Eskimos so healthy? The Inuit Eskimo diet is very high in fat, and yet Eskimos have a low incidence of heart disease, high cholesterol levels, and hypertension. Not surprisingly, much of the dietary fat they consume comes from fish rich in omega-3s.

One study involved 11,324 patients who had just survived a heart attack. They were randomly assigned supplements of omega-3 oils (1 g daily), vitamin E (300 mg daily), both, or none. Researchers found that omega-3 supplementation, but not vitamin E, lowered the risk of death, heart attack, and stroke. They concluded, "Dietary supplementation with n-3 polyunsaturated fatty acids led to a clinically important and statistically significant benefit."[38]

In a review of this study, the authors conclude that relatively small intakes of omega-3 fatty acids may work by stabilizing the heart muscle itself.[39]

How Much Omega-3 Is Recommended?

Omega-3 oils supply eicosapentaenoic acid (EPA) and docosahexaenoic acid (DHA). These two compounds protect against dangerous blood clotting, reduce triglyceride levels, and increase levels of HDL cholesterol. This is why mainstream medicine recommends two or three servings per week of fish, which provides a wealth of omega-3 fatty acids.

Symptoms of an essential fatty acid deficiency or imbalance include fatigue, dry skin, cracked nails, constipation, impaired immune function, aching joints, lack of motivation, and forgetfulness.

There is no recommended dietary allowance (RDA) for omega-3s. Six to 9 grams per week appears to be beneficial.

Omega-3 oils are highly unsaturated, and that means they are especially susceptible to oxidation. Once they become rancid, they can do more harm than good. For that reason, keep your omega-3 oils refrigerated and make sure your diet is rich in antioxidants such as vitamins C and E.

Omega-3 fatty acids help thin the blood. If you are already taking blood-thinning medication, speak to your doctor before taking supplemental omega-3s. In addition, women who menstruate may face a greater risk of anemia if they are ingesting large amounts of omega-3 oils.

If you are taking a flaxseed oil or fish oil supplement, consider taking vitamin E, too. Vitamin E is a fat-soluble antioxidant and protects against the chemical degradation of oils rich in omega-3s.

Good sources of omega-3 oils include cold-water fish, especially cod, tuna, salmon, halibut, shark, and mackerel. Other good sources are bluefish, shrimp, flounder, swordfish, and herring. A 7-ounce portion of herring provides 3.2 grams of omega-3s. Flaxseeds, flaxseed oil, and cod liver oil also provide high levels of omega-3s.

When adding fatty acids to the diet, make sure that all the companion nutrients are adequately supplied, such as the vitamin B complex and zinc. Zinc is required to activate the omega-3 fatty acids, as is the B complex. The average American only consumes about 5 to 6 mg of zinc daily, although the RDA is 15 mg.

Putting It All Together

How does all this fit together? Where do we start? How much of this do we have to take, and how do we take it?

The easiest way to meet the nutritional needs of the heart (after you are eating a healthy, well-balanced diet) is to select a high-quality multivitamin and mineral supplement that typically provides the following base nutrient amounts:

B complex (up to 50 mg/each)
Vitamin C (500 mg)
Vitamin E (200 IU mixed tocopherols, all natural)
Calcium and magnesium, preferably in a 1:1 ratio
Potassium (99 mg)
CoQ10 (see Chapter 7)
Omega-3 fatty acids (1–5 g/day)
Zinc (up to 30 mg/day)

Most dietary supplements do not provide all of these nutrients in these amounts. It may be necessary to purchase separate supplements, such as CoQ10 or the omega-3 fatty acids (flax or fish oil), to bring the total up to the recommended level.

Remember, They Are Supplements

We live in a culture that loathes deprivation and inconvenience. We would much rather purchase a bottle of supplements at the health food store and continue to indulge in convenience foods that harm the body and damage the heart.

The studies linking specific nutrients to benefits to the heart are often done in isolation from dietary changes. That is, indeed, unfortunate. Nutrients are not drugs. It is impossible to be deficient in just one nutrient because nutrients are always neatly blended in real, organic food. Foods contain vitamins and minerals, fatty acids, and proteins. When eating real food, therefore, the body is richly provided with the elements needed to build a healthy heart.

If someone wants to really study the impact of good nutrition on the heart, one should optimize the diet first, then add specific nutrients to boost the nutrient level higher, up to the level it would have been at the beginning of the world. Then we would see the benefits of good nutrition on the heart!

Until that work has been done, do whatever you can to promote the health of your heart. Eat food as close to nature as possible, and enjoy a wide variety of vegetables, moderate amounts of fruit and protein, and let the natural fats take care of themselves. Supplement your diet with the nutrients listed in this chapter. Chances are good that your heart—and the rest of you—will respond with new vigor and vitality.

CHAPTER 7

CoQ10: The Hero of the Heart

IF YOU HAVE BEEN KEEPING UP WITH the research over the past thirty years, you will have uncovered some exciting information about a nutrient that seems to target the cardiovascular system, reducing the risk of developing heart disease and possibly even healing the damaged heart. This nutrient is coenzyme Q10 (CoQ10), otherwise known as ubiquinone.

The research is truly impressive. Over the past twenty-plus years, scores of studies have confirmed the therapeutic value of CoQ10. Although CoQ10 is primarily regarded as a "heart" nutrient, it has also been investigated as an adjunct treatment for cancer, periodontal disease, neurodegenerative diseases, diabetes, obesity, and skin damage. Moreover, CoQ10 has shown to be beneficial in high blood pressure and other cardiovascular conditions.

Science and Serendipity

Science seems like a well-ordered enterprise to the layperson, but the truth is that some of the most exciting laboratory findings have been discovered quite by accident. One of these accidents happened in 1957 to a scientist, Frederick Crane, Ph.D. As Crane and his fellow researchers were studying mitochondria from beef hearts, they noticed yellow crystals floating to the top of a test tube containing fats from the mitochondria.

Crane became curious, scraped off the yellow substance, dried it, and looked at it under a microscope. The substance he was peering at through the lens was different from anything anyone had seen before.

Crane sent the yellow stuff to a colleague at Merck, Karl Folkers, Ph.D, (a highly respected scientist who had done outstanding work on the structure and function of vitamins B_6 and B_{12}). Folkers determined the chemical structure of this "new" molecule, a naturally occuring aromatic chemical from plants and animals, and began studying it in earnest in the late 1950s. Japanese researchers picked up the task in the early 1960s and began human studies in 1965. They were the first to use CoQ10 to treat congestive heart failure. Because of their (and Folkers's) work, scientists around the world began to notice the benefits of this vitamin-like substance for many types of heart disease.

What Is CoQ10 and What Does It Do?

Our bodies are composed of trillions of cells, and they all have one task in common: they must produce energy. Without energy, the cells simply cannot perform their assigned functions, and the energy of the entire organism (the body) wanes. Cells generate energy via a very complex series of biochemical events that break dietary sugars, fats, and proteins down into usable molecular components via enzymes and coenzymes. In other words, enzymes convert breakfast, lunch, and dinner into cellular energy.

Energy production takes place in an enclosure in the cell called the *mitochondria*. CoQ10, also known as ubiquinone or ubiquinol, is naturally present in our mitochondria, facilitating the production of energy and protecting our cells from free radical damage. The role of CoQ10 in the production of cellular energy is by activating the enzymes that help produce energy. CoQ10 is essential for the functioning of these enzymes..

CoQ10 is a fat-soluble nutrient. In tiny amounts, it is normally present in virtually all cells, but is more highly concentrated in the heart and other organs that require a great deal of energy.[1] CoQ10 acts as a coenzyme for many key enzymatic steps in the production of energy within the mitochondria.[2] (CoQ10 also performs as a very powerful antioxidant, protecting the membranes and other fatty substances in the cell from turning rancid.)

The body manufactures its own supply of CoQ10 within the cell through a seventeen-step process that involves the amino acid tyrosine, several of the B-complex vitamins (B_2, B_3, B_6, and B_{12}), vitamin C, and many trace minerals.[3] As might be expected with the standard American diet, inadequate intake of these specific nutrients may reduce the output of this vital molecule.

Vegetarians are often deficient in CoQ10, perhaps because meat is the best source of this helper protein. Vegetarian diets are also low in tyrosine, however, a deficiency that impairs the body's ability to produce its own supply of CoQ10.

According to the late Karl Folkers:

> Suboptimal nutrient intake in man is almost universal and there is subsequent secondary impairment in CoQ10 biosynthesis. This would mean that average or 'normal' levels of CoQ10 are really suboptimal and the very low levels observed in advanced disease states represent only the tip of a deficiency 'iceberg.' "[4]

If Folkers was right (and many nutritionists believe that he was), we simply do not consume enough "building-block" nutrients to produce sufficient CoQ10 to supply the energy demands of the heart and other tissues with high energy needs. Folkers's belief was that deficiency in CoQ10 is so widespread that we may not even know what a truly normal body level of CoQ10 is.

Other conditions leading to low levels of CoQ10 include the use of statin drugs (HMG-CoA reductase inhibitors) to treat elevated blood cholesterol levels. As these drugs lower serum cholesterol, they also block the synthesis of CoQ10 because CoQ10 and cholesterol partially share a biosynthetic pathway.

Since these two molecules share the same biochemical synthetic pathway, when cholesterol levels are high, CoQ10 levels are also high. Levels of cholesterol and CoQ10 run in parallel fashion. If this is true, as the studies show, when cholesterol levels drop on the introduction of HMG-CoA reductase inhibitors, CoQ10 levels drop only to "normal levels."

Randall Wilkinson, M.D., researcher on harnessing tocotrienols, part of the vitamin E family, for cardiovascular health, explains the parallel cholesterol and CoQ10 levels by stating:

> How does the HMGCoA (intermediate compound in the common pathway) relate to CoQ10 levels? It would appear that elevated mevalonate levels contribute to an increase in CoQ10 at the same time as they contribute to an increase in cholesterol. . . . But the question arises: is it good to have a boosted CoQ10 level at the price of having a concomitant boost in cholesterol levels (and, it would appear, cancer risk as mevalonate is a critical prerequisite for cell cycle initiation)?

People who are morbidly obese typically get more exercise than a normal-weight person because they're carrying around hundreds of extra pounds of weight. Indeed, their muscle activity can be pretty impressive. And since exercise is good and since the extra weight brings with it the extra exercise, then having extra weight must be a good thing—right? Well, we all know that is not true. There are other ways of getting more exercise and more importantly, there are other negative things that the extra weight brings with it. The conclusion is that one should get rid of the weight.

I think there's a parallel with regard to CoQ10. Although excess meval-onate (weight) brings with it a good thing—higher CoQ10 levels (exer-cise)—it's not necessarily a good way to get that good thing. So the issue of the excess mevalonate has to be dealt with as one issue (how to lower it). And the issue of good CoQ10 levels (how to increase them) has to be dealt with separately. Just as one wouldn't avoid losing weight because it was the source of exceptional exercise carrying it around, I'm not sure that one shouldn't be concerned with normalizing mevalonate levels.[5]

Dr. Wilkinson states that statin drugs normalize mevalonate levels that bring down the production of cholesterol. But he feels there may be safer ways of lowering these levels, without jeopardizing CoQ10 status, and theorizes that vitamin E in the form of tocotrienols may act as nature's own "statin drug," but without the side effects. More work is needed in this area, but as we noted in Chapter 6, vitamin E has long been shown to protect cardiovascular health.

Excessive exertion, hypermetabolism, and shock can also diminish blood CoQ10 levels, as can increasing age. By the age of seventy, we produce less

---

HOW TO OBTAIN COQ10

Foods rich in CoQ10 include organ meats such as heart, liver, and kidney. In addition, beef, soy oil, sardines, mackerel, and peanuts supply CoQ10. This nutrient is also avail-able in dietary supplements. Supplemental CoQ10 comes in the form of pressed tablets, powder-filled capsules, or oil-based gel caps. Since it is fat soluble, it is best absorbed when taken with food that contains fat.[6]

Numerous studies have shown that a specialized form of CoQ10 trademarked as Q-Gel is better absorbed than other forms of supplementary CoQ10. (For more informa-tion about Q-Gel, see the Tishcon.com website, or contact the Tishcon Corporation.)

than 50 percent of the levels that we need for health and vitality. Are we surprised that we are chronically tired?

The Mechanics

CoQ10 takes the electrons involved in energy metabolism and transports them within our cells, particularly within the mitochondria, explains physician and author Ray Sahelian. It is within these hundreds of thousands of energy-production factories that energy is produced from the breakdown of amino acids, carbohydrates, and fats.[7]

This nutrient is essential for the production of adenosine triphosphate (ATP), the body's main form of stored energy. Every cell requires a sufficient supply of ATP in order to keep up with essential functions. CoQ10 is like a spark plug. It generates the spark in the cells' mitochondria to help the body generate ATP and energy.[8]

CoQ10 has a vital role in the function of various organs and systems in the body. For instance, CoQ10 helps the heart muscle pump blood and is an important antioxidant, at least as significant as vitamins C and E.

Congestive Heart Failure

Aging, poor diet and lifestyle choices, viral infections, heart attacks, and stress can weaken the heart muscle until it no longer pumps efficiently. As the effectiveness of the heart is diminished because of low energy production or because of one or more of the lifestyle factors mentioned, blood and fluid can gradually back up into the lungs and every other part of the body. The supply of oxygen to the heart is also decreased, resulting in congestive heart failure.

Conventional doctors often prescribe digitalis, diuretics, or other drugs to boost heart function. Digitalis, derived from the foxglove plant, is used to treat congestive heart failure. Diuretics drain excess body fluids by promoting urination, thereby reducing the swelling or edema associated with congestive heart failure. These drugs are, however, often ineffective in treating this condition.[9]

One of the problems associated with the use of digitalis is loss of magnesium, a mineral that is essential to heart function. Magnesium works with calcium and potassium to regulate the heartbeat. Digitalis is associated with arrhythmias and other heart disorders, possibly because of the link between digitalis toxicity and magnesium loss.[10] Use of digitalis may also lead to anorexia, vomiting, diarrhea, and visual disturbances.

Along with draining fluids out of the body, diuretics deplete the body's stores of potassium, an essential mineral for heart health. Other possible adverse effects include weakness, low blood pressure, anemia, electrolyte imbalance, and muscle spasms.

CoQ10, however, is a promising alternative. One review cites the positive clinical results associated with oral CoQ10 supplementation, particularly for patients with chronic heart failure.[11] However, another study points out that more research is needed, and that CoQ10 is not recommended as first-line— or sole—treatment for congestive heart failure. On the other hand, these researchers state, "CoQ10 may be recommended as an adjuvant therapy in selected patients with CHF."[12]

According to one study, CoQ10 therapy resulted in a significant improvement in the "functional class (improved 20 percent), mean CHF score (improved 27 percent), left ventricular ejection fraction, and numerous other indicators of function."[13]

DEFINING HEART DISEASE

Classifications of heart disease, according to the New York Heart Association:

Class 1: No limitation in ordinary physical activity

Class 2: Slight limitation in ordinary physical activity. Patients are comfortable at rest, but ordinary physical activity results in angina, heart palpitations, or fatigue.

Class 3: Marked limitation of physical activity. While comfortable at rest, slight activity leads to discomfort.

Class 4: Inability to carry out physical activity without discomfort. Symptoms of CHF are felt even at rest. Increased discomfort with any physical activity is experienced.

One should not feel confident of "complete heart health" in the absence of symptoms, however. One of the first symptoms of heart disease can be a fatal heart attack!

The ejection fraction refers to the amount of blood pumped from the the left ventricle with every heart beat.

Not all CoQ10 research on congestive heart failure shows this level of effectiveness. But much does, especially studies in which serum levels of the coenzyme are actually increased to optimal levels.[14]

Heart Attacks

We know that blood flow to the extremities is extremely important, and that blood flow must not be interrupted due to clots. Unfortunately, blood clots can be a significant problem, especially for women who consume a diet that is undersupplied with vitamin E, niacin, and omega-3 fatty acids and over-supplied with cholesterol and trans-fatty acids (in other words, the standard American diet). Blood clots can also be a problem for bedridden or other-wise sedentary individuals.

Certain medications are used to protect against further blood vessel obstructions. These include (but are not limited to) heparin, beta-blockers, and nitroglycerin. Certainly, these medications may save your life. If your physician has prescribed anticoagulant medicines, you must not stop taking them without your doctor's consent. (See "CoQ10 and Other Medicines" later in this chapter.) However, they also have some drawbacks.

Heparin, an anticoagulant (blood thinner), is associated with hemorrhage, local irritation, chills, and fever. Prolonged usage of high-dose heparin may contribute to osteoporosis.[15]

Beta-blockers are a class of antiarrhythmia drugs that are associated with side effects such as new arrhythmias, fatigue, and elevated liver enzymes. They may also promote high glucose levels and greater insulin requirements in individuals with diabetes.[16]

Nitroglycerin helps dilate the arteries and veins by relaxing the smooth muscle of the blood vessels. As with most medications, adverse reactions are typically dose related. Side effects of high doses of nitroglycerin include headaches, light-headedness, low blood pressure, and rebound hypertension.

Here again, however, CoQ10 may offer an alternative. CoQ10 offers prom-ise in the treatment of AMI, or acute myocardial infarctions (heart attacks). A study of 144 heart attack patients explored the potential of CoQ10. For 28 days, CoQ10 was administered to 73 patients, while 71 patients received a placebo. At the conclusion of the study, researchers found less angina, fewer arrhythmias, and a lower rate of fatal and nonfatal heart attacks in the CoQ10 group than in the placebo group.

Furthermore, levels of beta-carotene and vitamins A, E, and C increased more in the CoQ10 group than in the placebo group. The researchers suggest that CoQ10 may provide rapid effects in patients with acute myocardial infarction. However, they caution that more and larger studies are needed to confirm their results.[17]

CAUTION!

Do not stop taking your heart medications without consulting your physician. If you are interested in CoQ10, speak with your doctor about how it could help, and the possibility of eventually decreasing your dosages of heparin, beta-blockers, nitroglycerin, high blood pressure drugs, or other medications. Abruptly quitting your medications could be life threatening.

CoQ10 and Heart Surgery

The heart, brain, and other tissues may not receive enough blood during heart surgery, resulting in increased levels of free radicals and subsequent cell damage.[18] As an antioxidant, CoQ10 helps protect the cells from harm.

CoQ10 may also be useful in certain heart surgeries. Types of surgery include (but are not limited to) cardiac catheterization, angioplasty, bypass surgery, and heart transplants. In a cardiac catheterization, a narrow catheter (plastic tube) is inserted through a vein or artery in the arm or leg. It eventually reaches the coronary arteries of the heart and is used to assess how much oxygen is in the blood and the blood pressure. It also provides information about the functions of the heart muscles, valves, and arteries. A dye is added, which makes it easier to find arterial blockages by tracking the dye flow as the treated blood passes through the arteries.

Angioplasty may be done during a cardiac catheterization. A small balloon is placed at a coronary blockage and blown up with air. This is supposed to compress the blocking material along the entire wall of the blood vessel. By inflating the blood vessel, the balloon ideally stretches the vessel so more blood can move through it.

Bypass surgery is recommended when severe blockages are found in several major blood vessels. Surgeons take a portion of vein from the leg, or an artery from the chest, and build a detour. This allows blood flow to bypass the blockage.

Heart transplants have also saved lives. Approximately 95 percent of heart transplant recipients find it considerably easier to exercise and take care of everyday chores than before the transplant.[19] These recipients must take immunosuppressant medication after surgery, to stop the body from rejecting the new heart. However, rejection does still occur in some cases.

A study of thirty-four patients after heart transplantation revealed a dangerously high level of oxidative stress and low levels of antioxidants. CoQ10 depletion was associated with this imbalance. The researchers suggest, "CoQ10 therapy could contribute to the prevention of rejection of the transplanted heart."[20]

Hypertension

Hypertension is increasing in this country, probably driven by a combination of added stress, obesity, increased coffee consumption, and lots of sodium. High blood pressure, or hypertension, has been called the "silent killer" because there may be no symptoms until a fatal cardiovascular event. More than 60 million people in the United States have high blood pressure.

Blood pressure refers to the force of blood traveling through the arteries. If the blood vessels and arteries are tense or tight because of mineral imbalances or other physiological situations, the flow of blood through the arteries is constricted, forcing the heart to work harder to get the blood moving through the arteries. Blood pressure is measured by assessing the number of times the heart contracts (systolic), and the rests between heartbeats (diastolic). Normal blood pressure is about 120/80. Borderline high blood pressure ranges from 120/90 to 160/94; mild high blood pressure ranges from 140/95 to 180/104; and severe high blood pressure is 160/115 and higher. More than 80 percent of people with hypertension fall into the borderline, mild, or moderate categories.

Doctors use a standard protocol for lowering blood pressure: lose weight, stop smoking, cut back on salt, eat more fiber, increase potassium in the diet, and restrict alcohol. It is excellent advice; these suggestions *will* help lower high blood pressure. Notice that all of these suggestions concern diet and lifestyle, not medication.

CoQ10 may also help with hypertension, particularly when used in combination with the above lifestyle and dietary recommendations. Several clinical trials have shown that CoQ10 supplementation can help reduce hypertension. For example, thirty patients who took antihypertension medication were involved in a randomized, double-blind trial. The first group took CoQ10; the second group took B-complex vitamins. After eight weeks of follow-up, the CoQ10 group showed lower systolic and diastolic blood pressure, less insulin resistance, and lower levels of triglycerides and lipid peroxides. In addition, the CoQ10 group increased its levels of HDL cholesterol, beta-carotene, and vitamins A, C, and E. All in all, several significant risk factors for heart disease were reduced or optimized. In contrast, the group taking B vitamins showed higher levels of only vitamin C and beta-carotene.

The researchers conclude, "These findings indicate that treatment with coenzyme Q10 decreases blood pressure by decreasing oxidative stress and insulin response in patients with known hypertension receiving conventional antihypertensive drugs."[21]

How does CoQ10 work to reduce blood pressure? This question calls for further research, but it appears to help relax the blood vessel wall. Resistance in blood vessel walls is implicated in high blood pressure and other cardiovascular diseases.[23] CoQ10 may also lower blood viscosity (stickiness), making it easier for the blood to pass through the arteries.[24]

Angina

Angina feels like the heart is being squeezed. Symptoms include burning, pressure, or an aching in the chest. The pain is mostly below the breastbone or in the upper abdomen, but it is also experienced in the neck, jaw, shoulder, elbow, wrist, and back. Angina is more likely to strike during physical activity, in response to emotional stress, following a big meal, and exposure to cold temperatures. However, when the arteries are narrowed by more than 80 percent, angina may strike at any time.[25]

An inadequate supply of oxygen to the heart causes angina. Typically, blockages in the coronary arteries are the reason for a restricted blood supply.[26]

Medications used for angina include (but are not limited to) nitrates, calcium channel blockers, ACE inhibitors, and anticoagulants (blood thinners). Nitrates are used to reduce the pain of angina and the risk of heart attacks by relaxing the smooth muscle and widening the arteries. Nitroglycerin is a common form of nitrate. Adverse side effects include diarrhea, anemia, drowsiness, facial swelling, and renal failure.

Anticoagulants, such as coumadin and warfarin, are blood thinners that reduce the risk of blood clots, especially after heart surgery. They are recommended for individuals with artificial heart valves, arrhythmias, and blood-clotting disorders. Potential adverse reactions to anticoagulants include uncontrolled bleeding, dermatitis, fever, nausea, and diarrhea.

CoQ10 may be an effective substitute for prescription medications, or as an adjuvant treatment for angina, with very few and very mild side effects. In an early double-blind, placebo-controlled, crossover study in Japan, researchers explored the potential of CoQ10 in 12 patients who had stable angina pectoris. CoQ10 (doses of 150 to 300 mg daily) was compared with a placebo in 37 patients. It was found that CoQ10 was associated with increased exercise duration and decreased frequency of anginal attacks. The authors concluded, "This study suggests that CoQ10 is a safe and promising treatment for angina pectoris."[27]

High Cholesterol and Atherosclerosis

If plaque is building up in the arteries that supply blood and oxygen to your heart, you are developing coronary artery disease. Like high blood pressure, high cholesterol levels do not produce symptoms, and it is easy to assume that nothing is wrong. But just as hypertension has been called the "silent killer," high cholesterol can also kill—silently lying in wait until a life event triggers an event. Again, a fatal heart attack may be the first—and only—symptom.

When the artery is extremely narrowed, the heart may not be able to pump sufficient blood and oxygen to the heart, brain, or legs. If symptoms do appear, they may include chest pains (angina) and leg cramps (intermittent claudication). Ultimately, atherosclerosis can lead to angina, heart attack, arrhythmias, heart failure, stroke, kidney failure, or obstructed peripheral arteries.

The statins are the most well-known medications used to lower LDL and total cholesterol and protect against atherosclerosis and heart attacks. *The Physicians' Desk Reference* (PDR) emphasizes that before using statins, attempts should be made to lower high cholesterol levels through appropriate diet (one low in saturated fat and cholesterol), exercise, weight loss in obese individuals, and the treatment of other, underlying medical problems. This is especially important because, as with the other heart medications, statins have been linked with renal failure and myopathy.

CoQ10 may be a viable alternative because it helps prevent the oxidation of lipoproteins—such as HDL and LDL—in the bloodstream. In the bloodstream, lipoproteins are mostly responsible for transporting CoQ10. It is believed that when LDL is oxidized, CoQ10 is the first antioxidant to become depleted in the body.[28] A study on rodents indicates that the combination of CoQ10 and vitamin E offers stronger protection against atherosclerosis than either one alone.[29] Another study suggests that CoQ10 reduces LDL oxidation ten times faster than vitamin E.[30] Peter H. Langsjoen, M.D., F.A.A.C., suggests that CoQ10 may benefit those with ischemia as well.[31]

CoQ10 Deficiency

So far, little has been published about CoQ10 deficiency. CoQ10 deficiency has been confirmed, however, in individuals with congestive heart failure, coronary artery disease, angina pectoris, high blood pressure, and mitral valve prolapse. CoQ10 deficiencies are also common in those undergoing coronary artery bypass surgery.[32]

It appears that the severity of congestive heart failure parallels the degree of CoQ10 deficiency. Researchers are still uncertain whether the CoQ10 deficiency is the primary or secondary causative factor.[33] However, some researchers suspect that CoQ10 deficiency contributes to most cases of heart disease. By addressing this deficiency, they speculate, patients can get their heart health under control.

According to researcher Karl Folkers, biosynthesis is the primary source of CoQ10 in the body. In other words, the body produces its own supply of this critical molecule. For many reasons, including inadequate dietary supply of the "building blocks" of CoQ10, or excessive demands because of stress or other lifestyle issues, we simply may not be able to produce enough, however. Folkers claimed that "normal" CoQ10 levels are insufficient to protect health.[34]

Folkers analyzed clinical studies of 110 Japanese heart specialists. These studies involved thousands of heart patients between 1967 and 1976. He concluded that blood and tissue levels of CoQ10 were substantially lower in individuals with heart disease than in those with healthy cardiovascular systems.[35]

Renowned heart surgeon Denton Cooley, M.D., has found significant deficiencies of CoQ10 in the hearts of 75 percent of patients with cardiovascular disease.[36]

As mentioned, cholesterol-lowering drugs interfere with the body's biosynthesis of CoQ10 because they share a common biochemical pathway. Other factors that may deplete CoQ10 levels are age, alcohol consumption, strenuous exercise, extreme cold, and illness.[37] Furthermore, deficiencies in folate; vitamins C, B_{12}, and B_6; pantothenic acid; amino acids; and/or trace minerals can lead to a CoQ10 deficiency.[38] Deficiencies in each of these nutrients are common and perhaps even to be expected in our dieting society. Women who have dieted frequently over their lifetimes often suffer from chronic malnutrition, a condition that will ultimately lead to significant health challenges such as cardiovascular disease.

It is also likely that chronic stress leads to a deficiency in CoQ10. Unrelenting stress places a huge metabolic burden on the body, raising the demand for cellular energy to compensate for the increased heart rate and blood pressure that accompanies chronic stress.

Symptoms of CoQ10 deficiency include fatigue and muscle aches. Unfortunately, most laboratories do not test for blood CoQ10 levels. CoQ10 testing calls for additional equipment and specialized employees not found in most testing laboratories and hospitals.

Because most of the CoQ10 we get through food is found in meat, vegetarians may not consume enough of this important nutrient. If you're a vegetarian, taking 10 mg of supplemental CoQ10 daily would certainly be safe and may be beneficial, states Dr. Sahelian. If CoQ10 deficiency is associated with heart disease, perhaps replenishing CoQ10 supplies will promote heart health. More research is needed, however.

What About Side Effects?

Occasionally, individuals taking high doses of CoQ10 have reported nausea, overstimulation, and insomnia. However, long-term use appears to be safe.[39]

How Long Should One Take CoQ10?

According to one published review, daily supplements of up to 200 mg of CoQ10 for six to twelve months yielded no reports of adverse effects. Furthermore, 100 mg of CoQ10 for up to six years appeared to be safe.[40]

A year and a half is the average length of time individuals take CoQ10. No side effects were reported, except for occasional nausea. Your doctor or nutritionist can help you find the most effective dosage. Dr. Sahelian recommends staying on the lowest effective dose.[41]

CoQ10 and Other Medicines

Dozens of heart medicines are available, including different types of diuretics (water pills), antiarrhythmic agents (to prevent heart irregularities), blood pressure medicines (calcium channel blockers, blood vessel dilators), digitalis, and others. Evidence suggests that lovastatin, a popular cholesterol-lowering drug, decreases the body's stores of CoQ10.[42] Zocor, Mevacor, and Pravachol appear to have the same effect. The latter three drugs appear to reduce blood levels of CoQ10 by 30 to 50 percent.[43] Of course, low levels of CoQ10 are associated with cardiovascular disease. If you are taking cholesterol-lowering drugs, talk with your doctor about CoQ10. When heart function improves with the use of CoQ10, regular medical follow-ups are recommended, with a specific focus on concominant medications. Stephen T. Sinatra, M.D., points out that the best antihypretension medicine would be affordable, work without side effects, and decrease the risk of cardiovascular disease, stroke, and kidney disease. He states that although there are at least seventy-five different antihypertension drugs now available, he has found none that meet his criteria. He adds that the use of CoQ10 is an integral part of his hypertension treatment protocol.[44]

The impact of the combination of CoQ10 and various medications needs to be studied further. Therefore, consult your physician before combining CoQ10 with any drug.

Recommended Amount

Since every patient is unique, it is difficult to recommend a one-size-fits-all dosage of CoQ10. Furthermore, congestive heart failure is a life-threatening condition, and close medical supervision is critical.

No recommended dietary allowance (RDA) has been established for CoQ10. Most people get 2 to 10 mg of CoQ10 every day through diet, unless they are vegetarians. In his book, *Heart Sense for Women,* Dr. Sinatra recommends a range of CoQ10 supplementation, starting with 60 to 90 mg/day to prevent heart disease and provide antiaging benefits to the mitochondria of the cell; 90 to 150 mg/day for Type 2 diabetes, insulin resistance, or a family history of diabetes; 120 to 240 mg/day for high blood pressure, angina, arrhythmia, mitral valve prolapse, and periodontal disease; and 300 to 400 mg/day for advanced congestive heart failure.

The definition of the "optimal dose" has gradually changed in the past two decades. Originally, 30 to 45 mg daily was linked to improvements in patients with heart failure. Today, 100 to 300 mg is recommended, depending on an individual's health and ability to absorb CoQ10.

CoQ10 is often combined with another nutrient, L-carnitine, an amino acid-like nutrient that acts as a shuttle to carry fats into the mitochondria where they can be "burned" for energy production. Dosages of L-carnitine range from 500 mg per day to 2,000 mg per day and can be very stimulating. There is some thought that the combination of CoQ10 and carnitine is not only protective to the heart and highly stimulating to energy-starved tissue, it can also act as an aid to weight loss. However, more research is needed.

Final Thoughts

The medical literature supports the value of CoQ10 and other nutritional compounds as adjunct therapies for heart disease. One review concluded, "Although additional intervention studies are needed, current scientific evidence generally supports nutritional supplementation with these nutrients (CoQ10; vitamins E, C, and B_6; folate; L-arginine; and proprionyl L-carnitine) as an effective adjunctive strategy for cardiovascular disease."[45]

Dr. Peter Langsjoen states, "The clinical experience with CoQ10 in heart disease is nothing short of dramatic, and it is reasonable to believe the entire field of medicine should be reevaluated in light of this growing knowledge."[46]

If CoQ10 is so effective, why isn't it commonly used as an adjunct treatment for heart disease? Sadly, its use is limited because of politics and marketing. Pharmaceutical companies can afford to fund research only on their own products. In addition, pharmaceutical medications can be patented, unlike natural substances. Those who study CoQ10 and other natural compounds must find other sources for funding, without any possibility of defraying their costs.

You are encouraged to do your own research on CoQ10 if you feel you fit the profile of CoQ10 deficiency. Speak with your physician, particularly if you have been using a statin drug to lower cholesterol levels. Your CoQ10 levels may be lowered as well.

Note: The ability of CoQ10 to prevent various illnesses has not been studied sufficiently. The research on CoQ10 focuses on its therapeutic impact on disease states. The discovery of CoQ10 was supported by the National Heart Institute and the National Institutes of Health (NIH) at the Institute for Enzyme Research at the University of Wisconsin.

CHAPTER 8

Nature's Medicine
for the Heart

WELCOME TO THE EXCITING WORLD of natural healing—and the world of herbs. The health food industry is a fairly new phenomenon in this country (developed only within the past fifty years), so it is easy to believe that herbal remedies are new. One could argue that we didn't need a health food industry prior to the industrialization of the food supply, the "better living through chemistry" concept, and our twenty-first century sedentary lifestyle. After all, until the turn of the twentieth century, many doctors had never treated a heart patient because they had never encountered one.

It should also be remembered that herbs have been used as food and medicine throughout recorded history. Hippocrates and Galen didn't use digitalis or heparin, did they? They did, apparently, use foxglove, from which digitalis is derived. Even today, in our society full of expensive, complex medications, much of the world still relies on ancient healing traditions that include local flowers, barks, leaves, and roots.

We use modern pharmaceutical medicines today, not because they work better or because herbs don't work. We use them simply because pharmaceutical companies market drugs to the doctors. They don't market herbs because there isn't a lot of money to be made on herbs. The question of natural remedies versus pharmaceuticals is a political and economic question, not a medical one.

While pharmaceutical firms would like us to believe that "drugs are safe because they are tested and the FDA has approved them" and "herbs are dangerous because they aren't tested and the FDA hasn't approved them," the truth is that when health-promoting herbs are used prudently and wisely, the risk of harm is small. Want to know how dangerous herbs are? Go to the CDC website and check out the adverse reactions to herbal products, then compare this data to the side effects and potential for harm with drugs. Herbs win the safety contest every time.

Of course, this is not to say that pharmaceuticals should never be used. Sometimes, drugs save lives, and when we address a serious health problem such as cardiovascular disease, we must discuss the treatment alternatives with our health care practitioners. When a drug is necessary to save or prolong a life, it must be employed.

However, lifestyle modification is still the number-one protocol for the prevention and treatment of heart disease. According to government statistics, up to 80 percent of all illness could be avoided if we made simple lifestyle changes. Part of these changes (in addition to a good diet, exercise, reducing stress, quitting smoking, and so on) can include the prudent use of ancient remedies.

Herbs can be marvelously protective—and healing—to the heart. Which herbs are specifically designed to nourish and heal the heart? Nature has provided a complex botanical armamentarium against heart disease.

Herbs for Heart, Blood Pressure, Cholesterol, and Atherosclerosis

Hawthorn (Crataegus, various species)

One of the best-known herbs in the treatment of heart disease are the flowers, leaves, and fruits of the hawthorn tree. The hawthorn berry is richly colored in red to blue with flavonoids that open the smooth vessels of the coronary arteries.

Native to Europe, hawthorn is a spiny tree or shrub that is often grown as a hedge plant, dividing plots of land. Hawthorn is "especially useful in treating the heart fatigue known as congestive heart failure," writes herbalist and author James A. Duke.[1]

By increasing blood flow to the heart, hawthorn protects against heart attack. Hawthorn extract has also been shown to:

- Fortify the contractions of the heart muscle
- Boost circulation to the extremities
- Disarm damaging free radicals

Donald Brown, N.D., author of *Herbal Prescriptions for Better Health* (Prima Publishing, 1996), writes, "Put simply, hawthorn and its flavonoid compounds make the heart a more efficient pump."[2] Throughout Europe, hawthorn is used to treat mild cases of angina. It appears to work by opening up the coronary arteries, thereby improving the flow of blood and oxygen to the heart."[3]

Hawthorn extract is also used to treat atherosclerosis. When the collagen matrix of the artery begins to weaken, more cholesterol sticks to the blood vessel wall, possibly acting as a bandage on the weakened area of the artery. One theory proposes that if the collagen matrix of the artery remains strong, atherosclerotic plaque cannot develop because the bandage is not needed. Collagen is the most abundant protein in the body, responsible for maintaining all connective tissue. The flavonoids in hawthorn have a strong "vitamin P" activity that strengthens capillary, vessel, and artery walls. Flavonoids help maintain collagen fiber in the blood vessels' walls and also promote coronary artery blood flow.[4]

A prime culprit in atherosclerosis is high total levels and high LDL levels of cholesterol. One laboratory study suggests that hawthorn has a profound cholesterol-lowering effect in rats. At the end of six weeks, researchers studied levels of total cholesterol and LDL cholesterol. They found that hawthorn tincture protected against cholesterol accumulation.[5]

Moreover, hawthorn exerts a gentle antihypertensive effect by widening the blood vessels, especially the coronary arteries. It also promotes healthy blood pressure through its diuretic action.

The flavonoids in the berries help increase intracellular vitamin C levels, shield vitamin C from oxidation, and help strengthen capillaries.

Hawthorn has been found to be extremely safe for long-term use. There are no known contraindications to its use during pregnancy or lactation.

Garlic *(Allium sativum)*

Garlic may be one of the most commonly used (and studied) herbs in the world. Its history goes back to the beginning of time, as a food to enhance flavor and aroma and as a healing herb.

The *Codex Ebers*, an Egyptian text dating from about 1550 B.C., recommended garlic for hypertension, headache, bites, worms, and tumors.

Sir John Harrington, in *The Englishman's Doctor*, wrote this poem about garlic:

Garlic then have power to save from death
Bear with it though it maketh unsavory breath,
And scorn not garlic like some that think
It only maketh men wink and drink and stink.

In *The Healing Power of Herbs* (Prima Publishing, 1995) Dr. Murray writes:

In 1721, during a widespread plague in Marseilles, four condemned criminals were recruited to bury the dead. The gravediggers proved to be immune to the disease. Their secret was a concoction they drank, consisting of macerated garlic in wine. This became known as *vinaigre des quatre voleurs* (four thieves' vinegar), and is still available in France today.

Our modern version of the brew might include macerated (crushed) garlic, rosemary, and other herbs infused into balsamic vinegar and sprinkled over greens as a tasty, healthy dressing. Yes, it "maketh unsavory breath," but it tastes so good.

The use of garlic is, truly, bigger than taste alone. Increasing evidence indicates that garlic benefits the cardiovascular system. This food/herb has been shown to reduce total cholesterol and to raise HDL ("good") cholesterol. According to one study, gelatin capsules of garlic oil have a greater benefit for women than for men.[6]

At least one review claims that garlic effectively suppresses the oxidation of LDL ("bad") cholesterol *in vitro*, or in the test tube. Oxidation is associated with the buildup of arterial plaque in the arteries. The authors write, "These data suggest that suppressed LDL oxidation may be one of the powerful mechanisms accounting for the antiatherosclerotic properties of garlic."[7] Furthermore, garlic may improve the elasticity of the aorta, thereby protecting against atherosclerosis.

Researchers speculate that garlic may activate the production of nitric oxide, which helps blood vessels relax. Garlic is also a natural antioxidant. In a placebo-controlled, randomized, double-blind study, ten participants took 600 mg of garlic daily. Researchers noted that garlic supplements exerted an antioxidant effect on certain lipoproteins. In this study, the susceptibility to LDL oxidation was reduced by 34 percent in the garlic-treated group.[8]

Garlic also exerts a mild antihypertensive effect. Naturopath and author Dr. Donald Brown suggests that this may be attributed to its ability to promote healthy circulation. Garlic makes blood platelets less sticky so they won't clump together to form life-threatening blood clots. Garlic also appears to help disintegrate blood clots that are beginning to form.

Garlic helps thin the blood, so if you are already taking aspirin or another anticoagulant, speak with your doctor before ingesting large doses of supplemental garlic.

Ginkgo (Ginkgo biloba)

The list of health conditions for which gingko has been used are impressive. They include cerebral vascular insufficiency (insufficient blood flow to the brain), dementia, depression, impotence, inner ear dysfunction (vertigo, tinnitus, and so on), multiple sclerosis, neuralgia and neuropathy, peripheral vascular insufficiency (intermittent claudication, Raynaud's disease, and so on), premenstrual syndrome, retinopathy (macular degeneration, diabetic retinopathy, and so on), and fragility of the blood vessels.

Ginkgo, a potent antioxidant, offers protection against heart disease. A laboratory study suggests that the terpenoid and flavonoid compounds in ginkgo may also reduce the risk of ischemia and reperfusion.[9]

As an antioxidant, ginkgo neutralizes free radicals that would otherwise damage the cardiovascular system. Ginkgo may also protect against arrhythmia, free-radical damage, and ischemia-reperfusion injury *in vivo*.[10] Reperfusion is the restoration of blood to a previously ischemic area.

Due to its ability to increase blood flow, ginkgo is especially beneficial for people with vascular insufficiency (for example, Raynaud's disease, also known as peripheral arterial occlusive disease). Another form of peripheral arterial occlusive disease (PAOD), intermittent claudication, is caused by an insufficient supply of blood to the legs due to a narrowing or blockage of the arteries (usually the result of atherosclerosis). The result is a cramping pain, usually in the calf, that occurs while walking or otherwise exercising. For some, the pain can make walking even the shortest distances agonizing.

If you are already taking an anticoagulant, consult your doctor before trying ginkgo. In rare cases, ginkgo has been associated with gastrointestinal discomfort, headache, and dizziness. If you are planning to have surgery, tell your doctor if you are taking gingko or any other herb. As a natural anticoagulant, ginkgo could contribute to uncontrolled bleeding.

Green and Black Tea (Camellia sinensis)

Green and black teas are well known for their impact on heart disease as well as cancer. They are also used to treat high blood pressure. In one study, researchers compared the effects of glutamic acid and theanine, an important component in green and black tea. They found that theanine decreased high blood pressure significantly.[11]

Tea plants contain polyphenols, powerful antioxidants. Researchers have discovered that green tea exerts just as much antioxidant clout as the renowned vitamin E.[12]

In a clinical study involving sixty-six patients, researchers investigated the impact of black tea on endothelial dysfunction. (Endothelin is a peptide that dilates the blood vessels.) The study participants who drank black tea improved their endothelial function, thereby dilating the arteries. An equivalent amount of caffeine exerted no impact on artery dilation. The authors concluded, "Short- and long-term black tea consumption reverses endothelial vasomotor dysfunction in patients with coronary artery disease. This finding may partly explain the association between tea intake and decreased cardiovascular disease events."[13]

A more recent article confirms tea's protective effect against the effects of nitric oxide toxicity.[14] High levels of nitric oxide are associated with hypertension.

Green and black teas do contain caffeine, and overconsumption may lead to irritability, anxiety, nervousness, and insomnia. Decaffeinated green tea is available, but its therapeutic impact is uncertain. One method of decaffeination—using ethyl acetate—removes about 70 percent of the heart-protective compounds in tea. The other method—using carbon dioxide and water—removes only about 5 percent. Furthermore, the studies on green tea have focused on regular green tea, not decaffeinated green tea.[15]

Asian Ginseng (Panax ginseng) *and* *Siberian Ginseng* (Eleutherococcus senticosus)

The ginsengs are another group of herbs that have attained nearly super-natural reputation, especially in the Orient where they have been cultivated and revered for many millennia. Ginseng is in a wonderful class of herbs that may help prevent premature aging, exhaustion of the adrenal gland, and diseases of the heart. We are just now putting the science together with the folklore.

Asian ginseng and Siberian ginseng have been used historically as general tonics. In recent times, Asian ginseng has been shown to reduce high triglyc-eride levels and raise HDL cholesterol in the blood. In addition, Asian gin-seng appears to reduce the blood's "stickiness," thereby reducing the risk of blood clots and stroke.[16]

Siberian ginseng and Asian ginseng have many overlapping features. One difference is that Asian ginseng has more ginsenosides (active constituents) than Siberian ginseng. Both ginsengs have been shown to slow down heart rate, increase coronary blood flow, and lower blood pressure.[17]

Nitric oxide (NO) relaxes blood vessels and regulates blood pressure. Gin-seng helps trigger the release of NO, thereby protecting the cardiovascular system.[18]

In addition, both ginsengs appear to balance blood sugar levels. By pro-tecting against, or treating, diabetes, these herbs may indirectly promote heart health.

Large amounts of ginseng are linked with ginseng abuse syndrome. Side effects of this syndrome include high blood pressure, euphoria, nervousness, skin problems, sleeplessness, and morning diarrhea.[19]

Phytoestrogens

Natural hormone balance between progesterone and estrogen is protective of the heart, so it is no surprise that rates of heart disease rise when a woman's production of these two hormones decreases after menopause. One way that estrogen appears to support the cardiovascular system is by improving a woman's metabolism of cholesterol and fats. Estrogen raises HDL cholesterol and lowers LDL cholesterol. Women live an average of seven to eight years longer than men, and one key reason is their hormonal protection against heart disease.[20]

Progesterone is protective because it increases metabolism, decreases water retention, helps normalize natural thyroid production, and increases brown fat thermogenesis. There is some controversy about whether estrogens are protective against—or increase the risk of—a heart attack. One option is to use phytoestrogens (plant estrogens), which are much weaker than pharmaceutical estrogen. Phytoestrogens bind to estrogen receptors, mimicking estriol, the "safe" estrogen.[21] Dr. Michael Murray suggests that plant extracts have a tonic effect on the female glandular system, and that herbs nourish and tone the female system rather than exert a druglike effect.

Because research on the use of phytoestrogens and other hormone-influencing herbs is scanty, we only speculate that normalizing hormones has a heart-protective effect. However, it is still a good idea to balance the hormones using natural alternatives. Dr. Murray recommends using a blend of herbs such as black cohosh and chaste berry to relieve menopausal symptoms.

Herbalist David Hoffman, author of *The New Holistic Herbal* (Element Books, 1995) recommends a mix of herbs that includes two parts each of chaste berry and wild yam, and one part each of black cohosh, goldenseal, life root, oats, and St. John's wort. He recommends substituting motherwort in place of St. John's wort if heart palpitations, high blood pressure, or tension are present.[22] (Life root is not commonly used in this country and may be difficult to find.)

So far, there is insufficient research to recommend phytoestrogens as a first-line defense against heart disease. We are only speculating that by normalizing estrogen levels, phytoestrogens may indirectly support heart health. On the other hand, certain phytoestrogens, such as soy and licorice, demonstrate a more direct effect on the cardiovascular system.

Presently, there is some question about recommending phytoestrogens for menopausal women with a family or personal history of estrogen-dependent breast cancer.[23] Women with a history of breast cancer or other hormone-dependent cancers are advised to discuss their options with a qualified health care professional. In addition, women taking hormone replacement therapy (HRT) are advised to consult with their doctors before taking phytoestrogens.

Here is more information about black cohosh and chaste berry, two herbs with which every woman should become familiar.

Black Cohosh (Cimicifuga racemosa)

The underground plant stem, the black cohosh rhizome was included in *The United States Pharmacopeia* from 1820 until 1936. In other words, it was used in mainstream medical practice as an herbal remedy for menopausal symptoms. Today, the German Commission E (Germany's equivalent to the Food and Drug Administration in the United States) approves black cohosh for menopausal symptoms, painful menstruation, and premenstrual discomfort. The herb is often sold under the brand name of Remifemin. Other companies also provide this valuable herb. Because of its estrogen-like action and relaxing effects on uterine muscle, black cohosh is not recommended for women who are pregnant or nursing.

Note: Large doses (well above therapeutic doses) of black cohosh have been linked to nausea, vomiting, headache, and dizziness. Long-term use, at recommended doses, appears to be safe.[24]

Chaste berry (Vitex agnus-castus)

Originally, chaste berry, from the Mediterranean chaste tree, was thought to suppress the human libido (hence its name). In fact, chaste berry appears to regulate, rather than dominate female hormones.

Throughout the centuries, chaste berry has been used as an effective herbal remedy for women's hormonal imbalances and has been shown to relieve symptoms of hormonal havoc, such as depression, cramps, mood swings, water retention, and weight gain.

Chaste berry appears to relieve menopausal symptoms such as hot flashes, night sweats, insomnia, vaginal dryness, breast tenderness, dry skin, headaches, irritability, and depression. This herb is believed to work by stabilizing the pituitary gland and progesterone levels. It is widely used in Europe to relieve the hot flashes associated with menopause and perimenopause.

This herb provides a wealth of flavonoids, antioxidants that protect against free radical damage and lipid peroxidation. They support the synthesis of collagen and strengthen the capillaries. Flavonoids are also natural blood thinners.[25]

Chaste berry is not a "quick fix"; it is a slow-acting herb. It is not recommended for women who are pregnant or who are using hormone replacement therapy. Side effects are rare, but some women taking chaste berry may experience minor gastrointenstinal disturbances or a mild skin rash with itching.

Soybean (Glycine max)

Soy is a popular herb/food/nutraceutical for women in midlife. Soy appears to promote heart health, along with many other aspects of health. Low rates of heart disease are found in countries with a high consumption of soy.

In fact, on October 26, 1999, the Food and Drug Administration (FDA) allowed food products containing soy protein to carry a label promoting soy's benefits for heart health. Foods that contain at least 6.25 g of soy protein per serving are permitted to include information on their labels on soy's heart-protective properties. The effective amount of soy is 25 g—or four servings—a day.

The FDA stated that its approval was based on evidence that soy protein, in a diet low in saturated fat and cholesterol, may help reduce the risk of heart disease. These labels are applied to soy beverages, tofu, soy-based meat alternatives, and some baked goods.

Soy appears to lower blood pressure and cholesterol. One study involving fifty-one perimenopausal women explored the impact of soy on cholesterol, blood pressure, and vasomotor symptoms (such as rapid heartbeat). After six weeks, the researchers found that the women on the soy diet significantly improved cholesterol levels, blood pressure, and perceived severity of vasomotor symptoms.

"The addition of even small amounts of isoflavone-containing foods to the Western diet may reduce the risk of heart disease," the authors of the study reported.[26]

Another study focused on the effect of soy isoflavones on the oxidation of LDL cholesterol. This randomized, crossover trial involved twenty-four subjects. Researchers found that soy reduced oxidation and increased the resistance of LDL to oxidation. The authors conclude, "The antioxidant action [of soy isoflavones] may be significant in regard to risk of atherosclerosis [and] cardiovascular disease in general."[27]

Controversy Not everyone is in agreement, however, with these findings, and a considerable amount of controversy is brewing about the new emphasis on soy and soy-based products. Naysayers point out that soy contains a considerable amount of phytoestrogens, enough to wield a potent influence on normal hormone levels. If a woman is already estrogen dominant or on hormone replacement therapy, soy may increase the estrogen dominance. (Another interesting question is, should men be consuming soy, thus increasing their levels of estrogen?)

Critics also cite literature showing that soy is one of the top ten allergens in the world, that it blocks the absorption of key minerals such as calcium and zinc, and that it is goitrogenic (that is, causes hypothyroidism).

Until these questions are resolved, it is prudent to steer clear of large amounts of soy, especially highly processed, genetically modified (GMO) soy products such as soy protein drinks and bars. Whatever the end result of the research, the present forms of soy (such as soy powders) were certainly never part of the food supply until the past few years. They cannot be considered a natural food, even if they are sold in health food stores and touted to be "all natural." A better choice is to consume tofu and tempeh made from non-GMO soybeans, as well as the whole cooked beans themselves.

Licorice Root (Glycyrrhiza glabra)

Licorice root provides estrogen-balancing compounds. These compounds appear to decrease estrogen levels in women when they're too high, and increase levels when they're too low.

A study on mice explored the impact of glabridin, an isoflavone derived from licorice root, on the oxidation of LDL cholesterol. The researchers found that glabridin, an antioxidant, appears to block the formation of lipid peroxides, thereby protecting LDL cholesterol from oxidation. By this action, glabridin helps inhibit the development of atherosclerosis.[28]

In another study, licorice was found to not only help prevent LDL oxidation but to protect the body's stores of carotenoids, which are also powerful antioxidants.[29]

Licorice root is not recommended for individuals with high blood pressure or kidney failure, those who use digitalis medications, or pregnant women. Furthermore, do not take licorice if you have chronic hepatitis, cirrhosis, or any condition that blocks the flow of bile from the liver. Avoid licorice if you have impaired kidney function or low potassium levels.

The glycyrrhizic acid in licorice has been implicated in high blood pressure and water retention in some people. It can increase the loss of potassium and sodium caused by diuretics. Fortunately, a safer version is available: deglycyrrhizinated licorice (DGL). Adverse side effects of licorice are rarely noted at intake levels below 100 mg of glycyrrhizin per day.

Herbs for the Emotions

St. John's Wort (Hypericum perforatum)

St. John's wort is not known for any direct health-boosting benefits for the cardiovascular system. However, as a natural mood booster, St. John's wort may alleviate depression, an important risk factor for heart disease.

In 1996, St. John's wort burst on the scene and took the country by storm. Until the media got wind of the traditional use for this common roadside plant and spread the word about its ability to relieve mild to moderate depression, no one really knew how common depression is. Many people who struggle with frequent bouts of depression never seek medical help; they simply suffer in silence.

The St. John's wort phenomenon opened a national dialogue on the "common cold" of mental health and whether people should be self-medicating with an herb or go directly to pharmaceuticals.

St. John's wort is believed to exert a positive influence on serotonin, dopamine, and norepinephrine levels. These neurotransmitters have a powerful impact, elevating the mood and relieving depression.

A meta-analysis published in the *British Medical Journal* in 1996 is what drew enormous attention to St. John's wort. The authors of this analysis thoroughly reviewed previously published studies, pooled the results, and concluded that St. John's wort was superior to placebo and *as effective as a pharmaceutical antidepressant*—and with fewer side effects.[30]

St. John's wort may also be effective in treating some cases of severe depression. A six-week clinical trial compared the effect of St. John's wort and imipramine, a widely used antidepressant, on severe depression. St. John's wort was shown to work just as well as imipramine. Furthermore, St. John's wort doesn't have the side effects of imipramine and other pharmaceutical antidepressants, including dry mouth, stomach upset, dizziness, and reduced sex drive. However, the authors suggest that "more studies of this type must be performed before a stronger recommendation can be made."[31]

New research suggests that the hyperforin component of St. John's wort has the greatest effect on depression.[32] In one laboratory study, hyperforin was shown to block the reuptake of serotonin, norepinephrine, and dopamine. Because their reuptake is blocked, these important chemicals remain available in the brain for mood regulation.[33]

Just as pharmaceutical medications don't work for everyone, St. John's wort only benefits about two-thirds of the people who try it. If you're in the one-third minority, you'll need to seek other forms of treatment.

In addition, be aware of the possible drawbacks of St. John's wort:

- Although St. John's wort has been proven effective for mild to moderate depression, the jury is still out regarding its impact on severe depression. Always consult a qualified health care practitioner for a professional diagnosis and treatment plan.
- Unless a medical professional is monitoring your condition, do not combine St. John's wort with another antidepressant.
- Until we know more about St. John's wort, it is not recommended for pregnant or breast-feeding women.
- St. John's wort can make the skin more sun sensitive. Fair-skinned individuals who take this herb should restrict their exposure to strong sunlight, tanning beds, and other sources of ultraviolet light.
- Nausea, loss of appetite, and abdominal pains are a few possible side effects of St. John's wort.
- Skin rashes and itching are occasionally reported.
- Rarely, anxiety has been reported by people taking St. John's wort. After the first few weeks of use, this symptom typically goes away.[34]

Kava (Piper methysticum)

The root of the kava tree has been used in ceremonies by the Pacific islanders for thousands of years and is highly regarded as a calming potion, much as we would consider an after-dinner glass of wine to be a calming beverage.

Kava has become a popular antistress remedy. It appears to promote relaxation, decrease muscle tension, instill a sense of contentment, and enhance sociability.[35]

Kava is not just for the mood, however. It is useful to the heart, as well. Kavain, one of the constituents of kava, may help thin the blood, thereby reducing the risk of blood clots and stroke.[36] An animal study suggests that kava may also protect against brain damage caused by ischemia, but more research is needed.[37]

Large doses of kava are associated with a scaly rash and eye irritation. Even larger doses may adversely affect the liver, heart, and lungs.[38] Individuals who are allergic to kava may experience temporary trouble with their vision. Do not combine kava with alcohol, other sedatives, or sleep medications.

Note: The Food and Drug Administration (FDA) issued a warning in March 2002 about kava's impact on the liver. It is true that kava leaves and stems are potentially dangerous and should not be used in kava products. Scientists at the University of Hawaii reportedly found a harmful alkaloid in some kava extracts from Europe, which included the leaves and part of the stem. For two thousand years, people throughout the Pacific have used kava root with very few problems, however. When purchasing a kava product, make sure it contains kava root and not its leaves or stems.

Herbs for the Heart and Herbs for the Mind

This is a brief overview of some of the more traditional and well-researched herbs. It doesn't touch on the vast library of information on the traditional use and the scientific validation of herbs, a library that is growing in breadth and depth each day. It certainly doesn't address the wealth of traditional knowledge, knowledge that has been passed from generation to generation for many millennia.

In our quest for information based on the "scientific method," we must be careful that we don't lose respect for traditional wisdom. Just because researchers haven't performed enough studies or produced enough empirical knowledge gleaned via the scientific method to satisfy their insatiable quest for "pure science," doesn't mean the value isn't there. The application of the scientific method may not prove to be the only way to study herbs.

Herbal medicines should be used in their traditional sense, not as "natural allopathics." Allopathic medicine is a form of medical philosophy that treats an illness with a pill—the "pill for every ill" mentality. It ignores the cause of the problem. It forgets that the body is a holistic organism and must be treated in a holistic manner.

It is tempting to use herbs allopathically in our quick-fix society. "Got this problem? Take this herbal pill . . . or take this herbal tincture." Even if herbs are safer than drugs, an allopathic approach is not the way to go.

Herbs fit into the holistic framework as part of prevention or part of the treatment, in partnership with dietary and lifestyle changes. Herbs are to be used prudently, carefully, and wisely. As such, they can help heal and restore the female heart.

CHAPTER 9

Tune Up the Whole Body

A S MUCH AS WOMEN HATE GIVING UP their favorite foods such as chocolate and doughnuts to achieve their health goals, they hate exercise even more. Women just don't like to sweat.

Exercise is uncomfortable. Women who are large breasted detest the feeling of "instability in the front region" when they walk briskly or jog. They hate wearing those corsetlike bras to keep them from bobbing up and down. Women who are large in the posterior hate how they look in workout shorts. Let's face it: whoever invented spandex shouldn't have!

We have been exposed to the shame-producing sight of buff women working out on those wretched exercise machines on TV. They have the audacity to smile as though their thighs weren't screaming. No sweat trickles down their happy faces. No bulges show beneath their spandex shorts. No rolls of midriff escape from under their crop tops. Where do they get these women?

That isn't us, is it? Few of us can relate to a woman who can handle that ski-like contraption without falling off. Unfortunately, no preventive health program is complete without an exercise plan. We're just going to have to get up off the couch and exercise.

One hundred years ago, the exercise movement didn't exist—there was no need for it. Women got plenty of exercise as they scrubbed their floors, plowed the back forty acres with a mule, or pounded their clothes against a rock in the river. They may have been a little heavy, according to our twenty-first century aesthetic standards (just look at the paintings of the masters in the seventeeth and eighteenth centuries), but they had muscles under those flouncy dresses. Physical labor was part of everyday life, before automatic washing machines, dishwashers, vacuum cleaners, and remote-controlled TV.

But now, if we are going to maintain a healthy heart (and a healthy weight), we must build exercise into our daily lives. We just aren't going to get healthy otherwise.

Exercise is critically important to a healthy heart. It is just as important to a heart that has already been weakened by cardiovascular disease. This is relatively new advice, however. As little as thirty years ago, women and men with heart disease were warned against physical activity. Doctors thought too much exercise would overexert an already weakened heart. Bed rest was highly recommended to the recovering heart patient.

Since then, the medical community has reversed its position. Researchers and health care professionals are realizing that exercise helps alleviate most of the key risk factors for heart disease: high blood pressure, high blood cholesterol, excess body fat, and diabetes. Exercise is also an effective treatment for many types of depression, another significant risk factor for heart disease.

How much exercise is required to satisfy the needs of the heart? Fortunately, we don't have to participate in iron women competitions or cross-country marathons to confer the benefits of exercise to our hearts. We just have to work out "a little." The recommended level of exercise is thirty minutes or more of moderate-intensity physical activity on most, if not all, days of the week. Or if you prefer, twenty or more minutes of vigorous-intensity physical activity at least three days a week will achieve the same benefits.

Research Supports Exercise Benefits

Researchers at the University of Minnesota School of Public Health tracked more than 40,000 postmenopausal Iowa women for seven years. At the conclusion of the study, researchers found that postmenopausal women who exercised moderately, *as little as once a week*, were 24 percent less likely to die prematurely than women who did not exercise. Activities such as bowling, golf, and gardening were considered moderate exercise.

The risk of premature death was 43 percent lower, however, in women who engaged in vigorous exercise, such as jogging, swimming, and other aerobic activities, more than four times a week.[1]

Aerobic exercise (any activity that increases the heart rate) includes running, swimming, brisk walking, aerobic dancing, bicycling, in-line skating, cross-country skiing, or even strenuous housecleaning or yard work.

The study also indicated benefits for women who didn't start exercising until midlife. The late bloomers had a lower risk of heart attack and heart-related death than their "couch potato" counterparts.

Exercise and Stroke

Consistent physical activity also decreases the risk of stroke. In the Nurses' Health Study, more than 72,000 female nurses, aged forty to sixty-five years, filled out detailed physical activity questionnaires in 1986, 1988, and 1992. At the beginning of the study, the nurses were healthy. They did not have diagnosed cardiovascular disease or cancer.

During eight years of follow-up, researchers documented 407 strokes—mostly among women who were sedentary. Nurses who enjoyed brisk striding or walking reduced their risk of stroke. While casual or average walking pace was good, it didn't necessarily help prevent stroke. The women had to work up a sweat! If they exercised frequently, the benefits accrued even more.[2]

Long-Term Effects

We know that the benefits of exercise accumulate over time. In other words, the longer and more consistently we enjoy our workout program, the greater the benefits.

We keep depositing exercise into our physical health program, and we build muscles all over our bodies. The muscles are metabolically active so they burn more calories, helping us achieve our weight goals. Increased muscle density makes working out easier and more enjoyable, so we engage in even more exercise, which benefits us even more! We *feel* like being more active. And our hearts just keep getting stronger. It's like compounding interest. What a deal!

How Does Exercise Benefit the Heart?

One way that exercise may protect against heart disease is through its balancing effect on blood pressure, regardless of a person's weight.

Aerobic exercise, at least thirty minutes three times a week, has been shown to effectively prevent high blood pressure by dilating the arteries, veins, and capillaries in the body, thereby decreasing resistance to blood flow.

Second, exercise is good for cholesterol levels. Following a moderate aerobic program of twenty to thirty minutes, four to five times per week, appears to balance out the bad (LDL) and good (HDL) cholesterol. Lifting weights (anaerobic exercise) for half an hour, twice a week, is also recommended for lowering cholesterol.

Furthermore, consistent physical activity reduces the workload of the heart by conditioning it to pump more efficiently. A good exercise program not only builds biceps, triceps, and "pecs"—it trains the heart muscle so it doesn't have to work as hard to pump blood throughout the body. It doesn't have to pump as many beats per minutes to do its job, which reduces its workload. In addition, exercise enhances circulation. In fact, physical activity is highly recommended for people who are concerned about varicose veins.

The Impact of Exercise on Coexisting Conditions

We know that coexisting illnesses can promote heart disease. Physical activity can indirectly support heart health by directly treating these other conditions.

Diabetes

People with diabetes are two to four times more likely than others to develop heart disease or experience a stroke, according to the American Diabetes Association. Diabetes is increasing rapidly in our sugar-loving, processed fat–loving culture.

Exercise, however, can reverse the grim prognosis of diabetes in the following ways:

- It helps reduce body fat. Excess body fat increases the risk of developing diabetes and its complications. Conversely, healthy weight loss can significantly improve the health of people with diabetes.
- It uses up excess sugar in the bloodstream, thereby balancing blood sugar levels.

- It makes cells more sensitive to insulin. Glucose is transported into the cells, instead of staying in the bloodstream.
- It increases blood flow, thereby improving circulation. People with diabetes and/or heart disease are especially vulnerable to poor circulation.
- It improves energy levels. Extreme fatigue is a common symptom of both diabetes and heart disease.

People with diabetes are urged to get a complete physical examination before starting an exercise program. Because of the potential for diabetic complications, a health care professional should check for any signs of heart, eye, kidney, or nerve damage. If these exist, the person with diabetes may need to alter the type and intensity of the activity.

Furthermore, people with Type 1 diabetes need to know that hypoglycemia—dangerously low blood sugar levels—may occur during exercise. Long periods of exercise are more likely to trigger hypoglycemia than exercise of moderate duration.

Physical activity can affect glucose levels for up to twenty-four hours. Individuals who take insulin should check their blood sugar levels right after a workout and again several hours later. They should speak with their doctors about their exercise programs and whether they need to alter their insulin intake.

Obesity

Obesity and excessive weight are contributing factors in high blood pressure and heart disease. Gaining as little as 10 to 20 pounds in adulthood increases susceptibility to hypertension. By the same measure, losing as little as 10 to 20 pounds of excess weight can lower your risk.

Out of more than 72,000 women enrolled in the Nurses' Health Study, about one in five developed hypertension. Researchers believe that about half these cases were related to long-term weight gain since age eighteen. Women who gained 11 to 22 pounds almost doubled their risk, and women who gained 50 pounds had five times the risk. However, losing weight decreased that risk.

Gaining weight early in life increased the risk of developing high blood pressure in middle age, and if the women continued to stack on unwanted pounds during their adult years, the risk ratcheted up even higher. But again, losing weight reduced the risk, especially in women who had a lot of weight to lose.

This really is a significant issue. Every 6 pounds over a healthy weight increases the risk of high blood pressure by 12 percent. (By the way, this appears to be true for men, too.)[3]

Exercise helps make permanent weight loss possible. It promotes the loss of body fat in three ways:

1. *Burning Calories*. This is where the research waters become murky. The body's way of balancing calories is much more complicated than simply adding exercise to a good eating plan to lose weight. Studies are very clear that while mild to moderate exercise benefits the entire body, significant weight-loss benefits don't follow until the exercise plan gets really vigorous. How vigorous? Well, it may require burning up to 2,500 calories per week to achieve weight loss.

   For those of you who aren't familiar with how many calories are burned during a workout, know that getting the exercise expenditure up to 2,500 calories per week requires working an intensive program for approximately one to one and a half hours daily, six days per week. That is discouraging news for many women—they'd rather stroll around the neighborhood with a friend.

   Here again, women—you'll have to sweat. However, the antiaging benefits alone from a vigorous exercise program make it worthwhile. Research is now appearing that shows that building lean muscle tissue to maximum levels helps reduce the aging process throughout the entire body. It also decreases depression—and lowers blood pressure and heart rate. How good does that sound?

2. *Metabolic Rate*. Your basal metabolic rate is heightened for four to twenty-four hours after vigorous physical activity. In other words, increasing muscle density and improving the muscle tone of the heart increase calorie expenditure throughout the day and during the night while sleeping.

3. *More Muscles*. Muscle burns more calories than any other part of the body. When you have more lean muscle mass, your body uses fat for fuel more efficiently. Your body becomes an effective fat-burning organism. Because fat is a dense source of energy, energy levels are improved as well. Every part of the body, every facet of the body's metabolism improves through a vigorous exercise program.

Just think: beside its benefits to weight control and heart health, exercise reduces your risk of diabetes and osteoporosis, relieves pain, improves mood and mental sharpness, and helps you sleep better. It promotes stamina, strength, and flexibility, and may increase longevity.

Depression

Depression is not just an illness of the brain; it is an illness of the whole body. We discussed depression in more detail in Chapter 4. Briefly, people who are depressed are more likely to develop heart disease or other physical conditions. One reason is that people lose their desire (or ability) to take care of themselves; they simply don't have the mental energy to stay healthy.

Exercise helps. In fact, consistent, vigorous physical activity may be just as effective as drug therapy. Physical activity triggers the release of the "feel-good" endorphins (pituitary gland hormones that function as natural opiates), increasing endorphin levels as much as fivefold.[4]

Exercise need not be strenuous to be effective as a natural antidepressant. Thirty-two elderly individuals joined a study on weightlifting and depression. Half of the study participants engaged in ten weeks of supervised weightlifting, followed by ten weeks of weightlifting without supervision.

At the twenty-six-month follow-up, researchers found that 33 percent of the exercisers were still lifting weights, unsupervised, compared to none of the controls. The antidepressant benefits continued as well.[5]

Multiple Benefits

Exercise increases the release of endorphins, but it also increases blood flow to the brain, pulling nutrients into the brain so it functions more efficiently. Aerobic exercise aids memory, stimulates creativity, and improves virtually every aspect of mental functioning. It also increases the release of certain hormones that influence brain biochemistry.

Exercise is a way of "exercising control" over one's body. People who work out regularly are generally happier, feel more alive, and enjoy higher self-esteem than their couch potato companions. There really is no part of the body that is not greatly benefited by consistent exercise!

Anxiety and Stress

Are you stressed? What woman isn't? Exercise may be the most powerful weapon against anxiety, a common by-product of stress. When you're experiencing anxiety, your adrenal glands work overtime to pump additional adrenaline. Exercise, however, burns off the excess adrenaline that would otherwise trigger anxiety symptoms. In addition, physical activity bumps up endorphin levels, also known as "feel-good" hormones.

Numerous studies have linked consistent physical activity to protection from the harmful effects of stress. One study focused on the impact of exercise on elderly adults with anxiety. At the end of the study, researchers found that after exercising, the study participants scored significantly lower for anxiety.[6] The key to successful stress reduction through exercise is to engage in an exercise program that you really enjoy, and don't overdo it. Exercise can, in itself, be stressful if the chosen activity is odious or too difficult.

Engaging in extreme forms of physical activity can raise adrenaline levels, worsening stress and increasing anxiety. But if you don't overdo it and enjoy the activity, exercise can help calm the nerves and focus the mind.

Too Few People
Are Getting Physical

With all this good news about the benefits of physical activity, one would think we would all be busily involved in exciting workouts. But the opposite is true; we really are a sedentary society. Seventy-eight percent of U.S. adults engage in less than the recommended level of physical activity, according to Micki Lavin, M.S., of the American Council on Science and Health. Sixty percent get no consistent exercise at all!

Why? We don't have time. It seems that everything is more important than working out. Busy moms put exercise at the very bottom of their "to-do" lists. Others find it too inconvenient. They don't want to drive to a club to work out—but walking can be done right outside the front door. Expense is another issue that comes up, but walking shoes are relatively inexpensive. Sometimes safety is an issue, but the major issue is, "I just don't want to."

Opportunities Abound

The first step in designing an exercise program that works for you is to choose a form of activity you really enjoy.

Meanwhile, you don't have to limit yourself to a formal exercise program. Get into an "active" mind-set. Here are some tips for increasing activity without going to the gym:

- Climb the stairs instead of taking the elevator. Start out with one flight of steps, and then build up as you become more fit. Take the stairs if your destination is lower than the fifth floor.
- Park a few blocks away from your destination and walk the rest of the way. If you're taking a bus or subway, get off a stop or two ahead of time and walk a few blocks.
- Clean your house at a faster pace. Better yet, sing and dance while you work!
- Mow your own lawn and/or shovel your own sidewalk. (Remember push mowers? Great exercise!)
- Carry your own groceries.

Got the idea? We don't need all these time-saving gadgets. We need to be more active!

Putting an Exercise Program Together

To build the health of your heart, your workout should include aerobic, toning/strengthening, and stretching exercises. An aerobic program should bring your heart rate up to 60 to 80 percent of your maximum rate for thirty minutes at least four times a week. (To figure out what your maximum rate is, subtract your age from 220, and then calculate 60 to 80 percent of that figure.) Aerobic exercise gets the blood flowing rapidly throughout the tissues, delivering oxygen more efficiently. Aerobic exercise lowers blood pressure, reduces heart rate, and strengthens the heart muscle. Include several sessions of aerobic exercise in your program each week.

Stretching before a workout reduces your risk of injury and muscle strain. Stretching increases blood flow, improves flexibility, and gets the body ready for exercise. It should be an integral part of warming up and cooling down. Several good stretching books are on the market; purchase a book and use it.

Strength training is also extremely important. Also known as anaerobic exercise, strength training increases lean muscle, which revs up the metabolic rate, which burns body fat. In addition, strength training improves balance, increases muscle endurance and mass, and reduces the risk of osteoporosis. Anaerobic exercise is often done with resistance such as weights or machines or bands. Carol enjoys working with bands because they are portable, and she can work most of the major muscles of her body with them.

Build up gradually. If you've been sedentary all your life, the prospect of getting active may be intimidating. Don't jump into it all at once. Take it easy at the beginning.

First of all, record how much exercise you are currently doing. Not doing any? Write it down!

Second, write your exercise plan. Can you begin with three workouts per week? Schedule these workouts on your planner, and keep the appointment as faithfully as you would any other meeting. Write it down in your exercise journal. Write a plan that slowly increases the number of workouts you do, until you are regularly exercising at least five times per week.

Third, add anaerobic exercise to your program. Remember the importance of building lean muscle mass? Schedule fifteen to twenty minutes several times per week, and work on all the major muscle groups of the body. (There are several good workout books on the market; purchase one and use it. Or consult with a personal trainer who can help you work out safely and effectively.)

Fourth, increase the intensity of your workouts. If you have chosen walking as your main source of aerobic exercise, increase the speed at which you walk. Or choose a course that has hills and valleys to provide more resistance. Make sure you are working up to your 80 percent level of intensity so your heart is getting a good workout.

Smoking and Heart Disease

In this day of increased awareness of the dangers of smoking, we probably shouldn't need to include a section on smoking in a book on heart disease.

BEFORE YOU BEGIN

If you're in good health, you may not need to see your doctor before starting a gradual, sensible exercise program. However, if any of the following are true, do talk to your doctor before you start or intensify your exercise regime:

- You have heart trouble or have had a heart attack.
- You are taking medicine for high blood pressure or a cardiovascular condition.
- You are 50 years old or older and have been sedentary most of your life.
- You have a family history of heart disease at a young age.

Also, stop immediately if you experience any warning signals. These include sudden paleness, fainting, and pain or pressure in your upper body just after exercising. If you experience any of these, stop exercising and call your doctor immediately.

The benefits of exercise typically outweigh the risks. However, there is a slight chance that vigorous exercise could trigger a heart attack, stroke, or arrhythmia. If you are at risk, it is critical to develop an exercise program with your doctor, especially if you have led a sedentary life.

We know, of course, that smoking leads to several forms of cancer, emphysema, and other lung diseases. However, smoking is also the single most preventable contributor to heart disease and other causes of premature death. Despite this, 22 million adult women and at least 1.5 million adolescent girls currently smoke cigarettes, according to the American Cancer Society.

Fortunately, smoking may be on the decline. The Centers for Disease Control and Prevention (CDC) reports that in 1965, 42.4 percent of adults in the United States were smokers. By 1997, that percentage had shrunk to 24.7. This decline has had a profound impact on the rates of death from heart disease. In 1950, 307.4 per 100,000 people died of heart disease. In 1996, only 134.6 per 100,000 people died of heart disease.

Although these statistics are quite promising, they still fell short of the nation's public health goal of decreasing smoking to 15 percent or lower by the year 2000.

The Impact of Smoking on Women

The National Institutes of Health (NIH) reports that women who smoke are two to six times more likely to experience heart disease than female nonsmokers. Every year, smoking leads to 34,000 deaths from ischemic heart disease in women. Every year, smoking is implicated in 8,000 deaths from stroke among women, according to the American Cancer Society. After the age of 65, women who smoke are twice as vulnerable to heart attack as men who smoke.[7]

Smoking more than doubles the risk of heart attack in both women and men. And when women combine smoking with the use of oral contraceptives, they are thirty-nine times more likely to have a heart attack than women who do neither.[8]

Constant Craving

Why don't women quit smoking? Once they have begun and become truly addicted to nicotine, it is harder for them to quit smoking than men. One study divided psychological from physical dependence on nicotine. Physical dependence was similar in both men and women, but women demonstrated a greater psychological need for cigarettes. For instance, they were more likely to crave a cigarette when they were out with friends or when they saw someone else light up.

The authors of the study hope that this insight will help in the development of smoking cessation programs especially geared toward women. The lead author, Thomas Eissenberg, Ph.D., stated, "Our work suggests that women who are trying to quit smoking may need to take care to avoid smoking-related situations."[9]

Smoking may be one of the most difficult habits to break, and many women who are otherwise extremely health conscious (and able to stop other unhealthy habits) believe they are unable to quit smoking.

What Smoking Does to a Woman's Heart

How does smoking affect the cardiovascular system? In premenopausal women, naturally occurring estrogens are believed to protect women against heart attacks. Smoking inhibits estrogens, thereby increasing the risk of heart disease.[10] Smoking also constricts blood vessels, thus increasing the risk of hypertension.

In addition, smoking increases the risk of atherosclerosis. It reduces HDL cholesterol levels and decreases the elastic properties of blood vessels, which slows down blood flow.

One study looked at the impact of smoking on atherosclerosis and lung function in elderly people. The carotid arterial walls were thicker in current and former smokers than in those who had never smoked. This thickening may lead to stroke.[11] In addition, the nicotine in smoke:

- Reduces the flow of oxygen to the heart
- Elevates blood pressure and heart rate
- Promotes blood clotting
- Damages cells that line the coronary arteries and other blood vessels

Even If You Don't Smoke

Even if you don't smoke, you may be susceptible to smoking-related heart disease if you live with a smoker. Consistent exposure to secondhand or "passive" smoke is believed to increase one's risk of heart disease by 25 to 91 percent. Many women were exposed to secondhand smoke as children because they lived in a home where dad or mom (or both) smoked, and for hours each day, they breathed their parents' smoke. Passive smoking (or secondhand smoke) can be just as harmful to health as if one were doing the smoking herself.

Impact of Marijuana on Heart Health

Tobacco isn't the only smoking-related risk factor in heart attacks. One study suggests that the risk for heart attack is almost five times higher in the hour following marijuana use.[12]

Let's Quit!

The good news is that the smoking habit can be broken—with help and perseverance. When the lungs are no longer forced to deal with smoke, they can be restored to health, as long as too much damage has not already occurred. Quitting smoking can reduce the risk for heart disease, as well as the severity of angina.

The American Heart Association recommends these steps for quitting:

- List all the positive reasons you want to quit smoking. Read the list daily and keep adding to it.
- Enlist the moral support of family, friends, and co-workers.
- Each day, try to smoke fewer cigarettes. Don't carry matches, and keep your cigarettes at a distance.
- Don't buy a new pack until you've finished the one you're smoking.
- Never buy a carton.

On the day you quit:

- Get rid of your cigarettes, matches, lighters, and ashtrays.
- Make a list of the gifts you'd like to buy yourself and others with the money you'll be saving.
- Get your teeth professionally cleaned to get rid of tobacco stains, once and for all.
- Stay busy: go to a movie, take a long walk, read a book, or enjoy a bicycle ride.

Soon after quitting:

- Spend as much time as you can in places where smoking is banned, such as theaters, department stores, churches, libraries, and museums.
- Drink plenty of clear water and fruit juices to reduce cravings and help flush the nicotine and other cigarette poisons out of your system.
- Avoid situations that may trigger the urge to smoke: watching TV, sitting in a certain chair, or stopping for "Happy Hour" after work.
- Keep your hands busy with toothpicks, paper clips, crossword puzzles, needlework, gardening, or household chores. Even snapping a rubber band may help.
- Find low-fat oral substitutes such as sugarless chewing gum, hard candy, celery and carrot sticks, or fresh fruits.

Natural Help for Breaking the Habit

Nature has provided some excellent tools for breaking the nicotine habit (and other addictions) in the form of specific herbs and nutrients. German medical doctor Rudolph Weiss uses oats to stop nicotine cravings. In his book *Herbal Medicine*, he writes,

> There has been much skepticism for some time regarding the sedative properties of oats. However, Anand published a report in which he describes how he learned about Ayurvedic medicine on a visit to India and found that decoctions of ordinary oats were used in opium withdrawal treatment. This led him to try the same method for nicotine withdrawal treatment. He prepared an alcoholic extract of the fresh plant and used this to treat a group of twenty-six people heavily addicted to cigarettes. Another group of the same size was given placebo. The oat extract gave clearly better results that were shown to be statistically significant.[13]

Oats (*Avena sativa*) are slightly sedative, but other properties of the herb may be responsible for its ability to reduce the craving for cigarettes.

Julia Ross, head of the Recovery Systems clinic in California, recommends two amino acids for nicotine addiction: L-glutamine and L-phenylalanine. Both amino acids work rapidly to diminish cravings for sugars, alcohol, and nicotine. For more information about breaking addictions, read Ross's book, *The Diet Cure* (Penguin Putnam, 2000.)

Alcohol and Heart Disease

Does alcohol help prevent heart disease? What about the French populace who drink large quantities of red wine and experience lower rates of heart disease? Is the alcohol preventive, or does it increase the risk of other diseases (such as liver disease, for example)? Research indicates that moderate alcohol consumption (one to two drinks per day) may reduce the risk of heart failure in older people or those who have already had a heart attack.[14] (One drink is considered 5 ounces of wine, 1.5 ounces of liquor, or 12 ounces of beer.)

A study in Australia explored the association between alcohol consumption and heart health. After adjusting for medical history and the effects of smoking, researchers found that women and men who drank one or two alcoholic beverages five or six days per week had a lower risk of a major coronary event than nondrinkers. The authors of the study concluded, "Risk is lowest among men who report one to four drinks daily on five or six days a week and among women who report one or two drinks daily on six days a week."[15]

The Mayo Clinic recommends no more than one drink daily for women, and two drinks daily for men. Women should be aware that drinking alcohol may raise the risk of breast cancer, however.

Confusion over Red Wine

Are certain forms of alcohol healthier than others? Again, looking at the research, red wine may be the beverage of choice for heart health. Red wine contains phytochemicals called flavonoids, which appear to raise HDL cholesterol. They also reduce the stickiness of blood, thereby protecting against blood clots. However, alcohol is not exactly a treatment for atherosclerosis, and it certainly is not appropriate for everyone.[16]

The flavonoids (especially the phenolic compounds) in red wine are powerful antioxidants, agents that disarm dangerous free radicals, which are implicated in heart disease and a host of other ills. Specifically, antioxidants protect LDL cholesterol against oxidation, or free radical damage. In addition, flavonoids appear to fortify blood vessels and shield them from free radical harm.

Resveratrol, another important compound found in red wine, grape skins, and grape seeds, is believed to provide estrogenlike benefits. Natural estrogens appear to increase HDL cholesterol. Tannins, also found in wine, seem to protect against blood clots.[17]

Is alcohol the ingredient that affects heart health? One study compared the impact of red and white wine, beer, and liquor. Researchers conducted a prospective study of coronary disease–related hospitalizations among 128,934 adults. After collecting data on drinking habits and health, the authors of the study concluded that all types of alcohol, in moderation, protect against coronary disease. Red and white wine seem to benefit both women and men, but beer may offer the most protection for men.[18]

Others believe it is the phytochemicals—not the alcohol—in wine that protect the heart. These health-boosting agents are also found in tea, onions, soy, and many fruits (including grapes) and vegetables.[19]

The Darker Side of Alcohol

Before we head to the bar in the interest of protecting our hearts, let's look at the dark side of alcohol consumption. It is apparent that while some forms of drinking may seem to be beneficial, the potential for overall harm from alcohol may far outweigh the possible benefits.

For example, is alcohol recommended for premenopausal women? It may be more harmful for this group, according to one study. "Among the young, the balance is negative, basically because the young drink more than the old, and because accidents and suicide are the more dominant causes of death," states Klim McPherson, Ph.D., one of the authors of the study.[20]

The American Heart Association does not recommend that people start drinking wine or other forms of alcohol to protect themselves from cardiovascular disease. Potential risks associated with alcohol include high blood pressure, irregular heart rhythms, weakness of the heart muscle, and birth defects in babies born to mothers using alcohol during pregnancy, points out Arthur Klatsky, M.D., in an editorial in the *Journal of the American Medical Association* (JAMA).

Another risk of drinking for heart health is that moderate drinking may grow into problem drinking or possibly alcoholism, according to Dr. Klatsky. Approximately 4 percent of adult women and 9 percent of adult men are considered alcoholics.[21]

It's important to keep in mind that alcohol is the second most widespread drug addiction, after tobacco.

Binge drinkers are individuals who consume nine or more alcoholic beverages once or twice a week. They face twice the risk of a cardiac emergency, such as a heart attack or stroke. Heavier drinkers are more vulnerable to accidents, colon and esophageal cancer, and liver disease. This is true of both women and men.

Final Thoughts

To sum it up, exercise is great! Smoking and excess alcohol (and marijuana) use are harmful! But we knew that, didn't we?

The challenge we face is putting this information to work in our own lives. Developing an exercise program is often postponed to a more convenient time (which may be never for many women). Stopping smoking may be likewise postponed until "our stress is less" (which is never). And who wants to stop indulging in that before-dinner glass of wine or two, or three? Wine is relaxing, isn't it?

As with any other health decisions, the biggest obstacle to making lifestyle changes is scheduling them into our day, making health a priority, and taking responsibility for our own good health.

Until some brilliant researcher invents a pill that replaces exercise (never), we're simply going to have to make exercise a priority. Follow the aforementioned suggestions for reducing the craving for nicotine. And by the way, if you are already addicted to alcohol or other recreational drugs, the amino acid L-glutamine is excellent for reducing those cravings as well.

CHAPTER 10

Healing Emotional Wounds Can Heal the Heart, Too

W E'VE DISCUSSED HOW EMOTIONAL HEALTH influences physical health, and we've certainly addressed how stressed (and unhappy) many American women are. We know that when our "hearts are breaking," our *physical* hearts are likely breaking as well. Can we also say, then, that when we heal our emotional hearts, we heal our physical hearts at the same time? Some interesting research shows that this may indeed be true. We cannot separate the mind from the body, after all.

Many of us listened to our mothers who tried to ready us for the harsh world. Our mothers typically wanted us to leave the safety of our childhood homes for the safety of a husband's home. Many of us grew up with no ambitions other than to be someone's wife and stay at home with the children while our husbands went out and earned the bread; we may not have considered any other choice.

The result? Years and years of internalized anger, resentment, unfulfillment, and repressed ambition. If our husbands dumped us for a younger, more interesting woman, we may have been left, in poverty, to care for ourselves and our children. Our hearts were broken.

These emotional breaking points affect our physical bodies. What happens when the social or emotional pressure builds to the breaking point? Women get depressed or anxious. They develop high blood pressure, or they have a heart attack.

We've seen that diet and other factors play a role in building the health of the heart, and we can't ignore any of these. Still, our emotional health is a powerful factor, and can tip the balance for either health or illness. Fortunately, there is much we can do to build our emotional health and confer health to our hearts at the same time.

A relatively new trend in medicine suggests that humor, hope, love, and prayer can work miracles that modern technology can't approach. Scientists have tried to measure the influence of these intangibles on physical healing and, given our scientific model, have found that they are not easily assessed. But rest assured, our minds are a powerful tool in healing the heart and the rest of the body.

Mind/Body Medicine

Thoughts and emotions can damage health; we know this instinctively. Even the ancient writings, penned hundreds or thousands of years before the Common Era, discuss the mind/body connection. For example, one author wrote, "My eye is wasted away from grief, my soul and my body also. For my life is spent with sorrow . . . my strength has failed . . . and my body has wasted away." Even the ancient writers knew emotional pain could lead to disease.

Anger is one emotion that damages the heart. Many of us live with years of unresolved, unforgiving anger. The Atherosclerosis Risk in Communities Study involved 12,990 middle-aged black and white women and men. Researchers kept track of their rate of acute heart attack, fatal coronary heart disease, silent heart attack, or cardiovascular revascularization procedures. Researchers found that an intense, angry temperament increased the risk of all of the above problems, even among the individuals who had normal blood pressure. They hypothesized that an angry temperament is as much a risk for heart disease as high blood pressure.[1]

People who face stressful events such as moving, losing their jobs, or getting divorced are shown to be at greater risk of heart attacks, as well as infectious illness or cancer.[2] But it isn't necessarily "bad luck" that causes the increased risk; it is the feeling that life is capricious and unfair. People who face trauma with grace and optimism do much better. According to *Learned Optimism* (Pocket Books, 1998), Martin E. Seligman, Ph.D., pessimists are more likely than optimists to feel helpless. Helplessness appears to branch out to the cellular level and make the immune system more passive, or helpless, Seligman explains.

According to Dr. Seligman, you are a pessimist if you assume the following to be so:

- The cause of your misfortune is stable and long lasting.
- The cause of a bad event will ruin many other areas of your life.
- You are to blame for the misfortune, rather than others.[2]

Pessimists are also more vulnerable to depression. But does powerlessness itself cause illness—or are unhappy people less likely to take care of themselves? Does it really matter?

Some People Attack Adversity with Food

It might matter very much, because two decades of research show a strong link between depression and harmful eating habits. Depression is often accompanied by appetite and weight changes, possibly because carbohydrate cravings are linked to serotonin synthesis. Serotonin is a calming neurotransmitter that eases depression, insomnia, and anxiety. Studies seem to indicate that depressed persons are deficient in serotonin, and serotonin release is increased by low-protein/high-carbohydrate diets. Cravings for sugars, then, may be its attempt to normalize serotonin levels in the brain to ease depression.

One author writes,

> Serotoninergic neurotransmission plays an important role in the regulation of appetite. Dysfunction of this system has been postulated to result in the clinical picture of carbohydrate-craving obesity. This subgroup of obese patients is characterized by a specific preference for high-carbohydrate and low-protein snacks.[3]

Other People Just Take Charge

If we can take charge of our thoughts and feelings, perhaps we can learn to take greater control of our health—whatever the route. Instead of eating a bowl of ice cream (and increasing our weight, which leads to heart disease) to deal with our depression, we take charge. We guide our fate, instead of allowing fate to dominate us.

Instead of lying down and giving up, some people face adversity with a sense of adventure. They take charge. They don't blame themselves or others; they make a plan. The authors of *Mind/Body Medicine* (Consumer Reports Books, 1993), Daniel Goleman and Joel Gurin refer to an "explanatory style" that distinguishes optimists from pessimists. They explain that when something bad happens to optimists, they are more likely to blame it on external sources such as fate or chance, rather than personal inadequacy. Optimists tend to view the cause of misfortune as short-lived and transient. Finally, they see their troubles as specific to one area, and don't expect them to spill over into other areas of their lives. In other words, they may occasionally fail, but they don't labels themselves as failures.[4]

Is it possible to learn optimism? More and more psychologists are saying yes. Cognitive therapy, originally developed by psychiatrist Aaron T. Beck and psychologist Albert Ellis in the 1950s, is based on the premise that our thoughts control our feelings. If we can adopt more positive habits of thought, we can make ourselves feel better. In addition, our feelings may "follow our faces." In other words, when we smile even if we don't feel like it, our emotions follow the smile on our face. We soon feel better, just from the simple act of smiling. What would happen, then, if we learn to think positive thoughts during difficult times instead of ruminating on our troubles? Could we change our physiology? Could we reduce our risk of heart disease?

One review pointed out that cardiac patients tend to be anxious or fearful about their life situations. This anxiety can diminish the quality of life by increasing symptoms such as chest pain and disability. Just learning new patterns of thought helps reduce chest pain.[5] In other words, they can *think* their way to better health.

Mind and Body: A Single Organism

Socrates once said, "As it is not proper to cure the eyes without the head, nor the head without the body; so neither is it proper to cure the body without the soul."

The mind and body are inextricably linked—in health and in sickness. In *Healing and the Mind*, by renowned news reporter Bill Moyers, scientist Candace Pert, Ph.D., asserts that there is no distinction. She reports that brain chemicals, such as endorphins, are found not only in the brain but also in the immune system, the endocrine system, and throughout the entire human body. Dr. Pert perceives emotions as the bridge between our mental and physical selves.[6]

The thoughts we think are converted into biochemical messages that promote either health or illness. Constant negativity (anger, unforgiveness, pessimism) are translated into neurotransmitters and hormones that increase blood pressure, heart rate, heart arrhythmias, and other physical symptoms. On the other hand, constant "positivity" is translated into soothing neurotransmitters that calm the blood pressure, and reduce the heart rate.

The stress response, brought on by physiological or psychological stressors, causes anxiety. When anxiety persists over a long period of time (decades, perhaps), the adrenal gland becomes exhausted or hyperactive, driving the levels of stress hormone, cortisol, higher and leading to an even greater physiological response. In other words, we train ourselves to respond vigorously to stress. We become "cortisol responders," pumping out cortisol (which elevates blood pressure and increases heart rate, and so on) over even the smallest of stress triggers.

On the other hand, we can learn a "calming response," just as we learned a stress response. We can choose to be optimistic and positive or we can choose to be angry or pessimistic. In learning positive emotions, we take control of our heart health.

Humor

Have you heard the one about Laughing Clubs International in Bombay, India? Founded by Madan Kataria, individuals in the laughing clubs get together in parks around the city of Bombay to do nothing but laugh. Sometimes they laugh aloud; they also laugh silently. Warming-up exercises include raising their hands above their heads, an exercise that gets the laughter started, and then the chortles and guffaws begin in earnest.

When did we adults get so cranky? Why don't we laugh more frequently? Maybe we just take ourselves too seriously. But humor is excellent preventive (and healing) medicine.

The late Norman Cousins was perhaps the most well-known advocate for humor and healing. In 1964, Cousins was stricken with ankylosing spondylitis, a painful disintegration of the connective tissue in the spine. He was told that his chances for recovery were one in five hundred. However, through nutrition, the avoidance of toxic medication, and the use of humor and hope, Cousins fully recovered from that condition.

In *Anatomy of an Illness*, Cousins writes,

> The regenerative and restorative force in human beings is at the core of human uniqueness. . . . One of the most important things a doctor can do for a patient is to assess the capacity of each individual to put that force to work."[7]

In fact, laughter offers physical as well as psychological benefits. Cousins found that ten minutes of belly-laughing gave him two hours of pain-free sleep. Laughter also reduces the stress hormones implicated in heart disease.[8] It lowers blood pressure, increases vascular blood flow, and draws more oxygen into the bloodstream, thereby promoting the body's drive for self-healing. When we're laughing, we're exercising the diaphragm, abdomen, lungs, and muscles in the face, legs, and back. If you feel drained after a long belly laugh, it's because you've gone through a vigorous aerobic workout!

Research confirms the health benefits of mirth, and conversely, the risk associated with humorlessness. Prior research has demonstrated a link between Type A (hostile, angry, impatient) personalities and an increased risk of coronary heart disease. In one study, the authors concluded, "These data . . . raise the possibility that the propensity to laugh may contribute to cardioprotection."[9]

Anger, depression, and a bleak outlook can damage immune function, but comedy displaces negative emotions. "Humor and distressing emotion cannot occupy the same psychological space," according to Steven Sultanoff, Ph.D., a clinical psychologist and president of the American Association for Therapeutic Humor.[10]

Another positive about laughter is that it brings friends and family closer to the heart. We know that a supportive network of loving companions is very important to mental and physical health. No one loves a grump! Remember the adage, "Laugh and the world laughs with you; weep and you weep alone?" Truly, an engaging person who enjoys a good laugh is more likely to attract a wide network of supportive friends.

Laughter is undeniably good medicine, for the heart and every other part of the body and soul. Isn't it wonderful to possess so magnificent a medicine that doesn't cost anything, that confers so much pleasure, that builds so many personal bonds, and that brings so much healing? Use it often!

Love

People were not designed for solitude. They were designed for relationships. In the context of healthy, loving relationships, the body and spirit remain strong. Study after study have shown that when women and men are bonded in a network of community, friends, and relatives, they are happier and healthier. They are also better able to cope with stress, and they're better equipped to resist emotional and physical illness. They also laugh more!

One study investigated social isolation as a predictor of mortality in 430 patients with significant coronary artery disease. Predictably, researchers found that the mortality rate was higher among the more socially isolated patients. The higher risk did not appear to be attributable to disease severity, demographics, or even psychological distress. The researchers concluded, "These findings have implications for mechanisms linking social isolation to mortality and for the application of psychosocial interventions."[11]

Dr. Seligman points out that people who isolate themselves when they get sick tend to become sicker. A study in Sweden investigated 292 female patients, thirty to sixty-five years old, who had been treated for an acute coronary event between 1991 and 1994. After five years, they found that women who remained isolated and depressed were more likely to die from heart disease and more likely to require coronary surgery. In contrast, women who enjoyed a vigorous social life became strong and healthy.[12] And when they did experience a heart event, they recovered more quickly.

Part of the love connection involves having a warm, intimate relationship. When a marriage is strong, for example, and the partners in the marriage provide intimate love and emotional support, blood pressure drops. The effect is immediate, not just cumulative. Studies have shown that blood pressure drops during "loving intervals." While friendships also provide benefits to the heart, the intimacy of a committed relationship provides even greater advantages.[13]

In *Mind as Healer, Mind as Slayer*, authors Kenneth R. Pelletier and Stephen E. Locke point out that people who feel they don't have enough social support are more vulnerable to high blood pressure and heart disease, as well as to arthritis and tuberculosis. Pelletier stated, "There is a link between disease and depression, loneliness, and hopelessness."[14]

On the other hand, just as loneliness can kill us, love can save us. At the Case Western Reserve University in Cleveland, researchers asked ten-thousand married men who had never had chest pains, "Does your wife show you her love?" The men who responded with a "yes" experienced significantly less angina over the following five years than the men who answered "no." These results stayed positive even after adjusting for high cholesterol, hypertension, diabetes, or electrocardiogram abnormalities.[15]

Here is where we need a similar study on women! If men consistently show love and support to their wives, will the women also experience less angina? Will their hearts be healthier, too? Surely here is no hormonal bias!

Fortunately, the folks at Yale University thought to include women in their small study of 40 women and 119 men. (Why more men than women?) These individuals volunteered to undergo angiography. Both men and women who felt loved and supported displayed dramatically less arterial blockage. Love and support helped preserve their heart health, and these findings were independent of diet, smoking, physical activity, or family history.[16]

Forgiveness

Some people never forgive, and they certainly never forget. Old grievances eat away at their souls—and their hearts—for decades.

It's funny how revenge tastes so sweet at first bite, but how bitter when it has run its course. This is how unforgiveness works. It doesn't harm the person who offended; it destroys the victim.

Bitterness (unforgiveness) eats at the heart; it actually causes heart disease. Carl Thoresen, director of the Stanford University Forgiveness Research Project and co-author of *Forgiveness: Theory, Research, and Practice*, says, "Resentment is the poison that you take yourself, yet hope the other person will die."[17]

How does unforgiveness affect the cardiovascular system? Grudge holding increases blood pressure. In one small study of thirty-five women and thirty-six men, researchers found that unforgiving people had faster heart rates and higher blood pressure. The authors wrote, "The results . . . suggest possible mechanisms through which chronic unforgiving responses may erode health whereas forgiving responses may enhance it."[18]

Forgiveness is not accomplished through one act of letting go. Forgiveness is an ongoing process, an activity that must be renewed every day. It must sometimes be practiced every moment. When the wound is particularly deep because the offender was a loved one, or when the abuse continued for a long period of time, forgiveness must be revisited every time the memory is brought to the forefront.

We don't simply *do* or *think* forgiveness; we *live* forgiveness. We get into the habit of releasing our judgment and anger on a daily basis so that bitterness never gets the opportunity to take root in our emotions and our hearts. When we choose to forgive, we lower our blood pressure and protect our hearts.

Forgiveness Is Easier with Age and Practice

Age and gender appear to influence our readiness to forgive. One study investigating 1,423 Americans found that people aged forty-five and older were more likely to forgive than younger adults. They also felt more forgiven. Eighty percent of the forty-five-and-older group believed that God forgave their sins, compared to 69 percent of those eighteen to forty-four years old.

Women are slightly more likely than men to "let bygones be bygones." Fifty-four percent of the women in this study scored high in forgiveness of others, compared to 49 percent of men. Forty-eight percent of women said that they had asked for forgiveness from another person, while only 37 percent of men did.

David R. Williams, a sociologist and senior research scientist at the Institute for Social Research in Ann Arbor, Michigan, stated, "We found a particularly strong relationship between forgiveness of others and mental health among middle-aged and older Americans." Forgiving others helps heal the heart—and it helps heal the mind as well.

Not surprisingly, we tend to find it easier to receive than to offer forgiveness. Approximately 75 percent of all the people in this survey believe that God has forgiven them for their past mistakes, and 60 percent say that they've forgiven themselves for previous wrongdoings. However, only 52 percent said that they have forgiven those who have wronged them, and only 43 percent have sought forgiveness for the wrongs they've done to others.

Not surprisingly, people who were more likely to forgive faced a lower incidence of nervousness, restlessness, or sadness.[18] It isn't enough to receive forgiveness or forgive ourselves. We have to offer it to others.

Spirituality

Prayer can have a profound effect on physical and mental health. Although our expressions of religion may vary from person to person, a relationship with God, however defined, can have a marked influence on physical and emotional health. Spirituality is intensely personal, but scientists have sought to measure it and explore how it correlates with health.

One study was designed to investigate whether scores measuring spiritual well-being correlated with either progression or regression of coronary heart disease. The participants in Dr. Dean Ornish's Lifestyle Heart Trial were given a "Spiritual Orientation Inventory," and considerable differences were found in the spirituality scores of a control group versus a group who practiced daily meditation.

After four years, researchers found that those with the lowest scores on spiritual well-being had the most progression of coronary obstruction. Conversely, individuals with the highest scores experienced the most regression. The authors concluded, "This study suggests that the degree of spiritual well-being may be an important factor in the development of coronary artery disease."[20]

Measuring spirituality may be technically impossible. What part of spirituality conferred benefits to the heart? Were the spiritual people more likely to forgive? Were they more likely to foster emotionally healthy relationships with others in their spiritual group? Did they pray more frequently or more fervently? Did they believe their prayers would be answered, that they weren't just sending words up into an indifferrent universe?

Part of it appears to be regular church, synagogue, temple, or mosque attendance. Researchers assessed the long-term survival of frequent churchgoers, compared with four widely accepted beneficial health behaviors: consistent physical activity, nonreligious social involvement, and avoidance of cigarette smoking and excess alcohol consumption. The study focused on 5,894 participants, aged twenty-one to seventy-five, in Alameda County, California.

For women, weekly church attendance appeared to offer just as much protection as the other healthy behaviors. However, for men, the protective effect of weekly church attendance was less than any of the other behaviors.[21]

Here again, the studies offer no clues as to why church attendance benefits women more than men. Did the men sleep during services? Did they take the spiritual counsel to heart? Did they develop intimate friendships with other occupants of the pews, or did they remain as isolated as if they had never gone? Did the men practice forgiveness? Did they forgive themselves and others? Did they pray?

Just warming a pew is probably not the beneficial part of church attendance! Praying is definitely a critical part of the spiritual experience.

Praying for Others and Ourselves

Scientists have always been a little skeptical of spiritual matters. God does not fit into a test tube. Spiritual beliefs cannot be examined using the scientific method. Spirituality seems far too subjective for a logical mind.

However, even science is now beginning to study prayer and is finding that it does, indeed, *physically* help to pray. Part of the rigor of the scientific method of study involves randomization and double-blind protocol. One unusual, randomized study involved nine-hundred consecutive patients admitted to a hospital coronary care unit. The names of one-half of the patients were given to a prayer group and the names of the other half received only the usual care. The prayed-for patients did not know they were being prayed for.

The prayer group received the first names of the patients, but did not meet them. They did not know the individuals for whom they were praying, but they faithfully prayed for them, by name, for four weeks. Researchers found that the patients who had been prayed for had fewer adverse events and a shorter stay in the coronary care unit.[22]

Interesting? Yes! Definitive according to the scientific method? Not quite. But perhaps it doesn't really matter. It never hurts to pray—and it probably may do a great deal of good—to both the recipient and the donor of the prayer.

Herbert Benson, M.D., founding president of the Mind/Body Medical Institute, studied the physiological changes that prayer could set into motion. He found that patients who prayed and/or meditated could elicit a relaxation response. Prayer slows the heart rate and breathing rate, reduces muscle tension, and sometimes even lowers blood pressure.

Furthermore, the slow breathing associated with the relaxation response may improve mobilization of the respiratory muscles, which may be helpful to those with heart failure.[22] Slow breathing lowers heart rate, muscle tension, and blood pressure.

What Now?

Speaking of matters of the heart and mind has become easier for us. Many of us are at ease talking about our emotions and our spirituality, and we are finding it less difficult to develop a healing network of friends.

Additionally, the medical community is no longer squeamish about discussing matters of the heart with their patients. Humor rooms have cropped up in hospitals across the country, complete with games, movies, magazines, and funny books. In most hospitals, rigid visiting hours are an outdated concept, as health care professionals begin to recognize the healing impact of companionship. They want family and friends to visit often because they know that love is a great healer.

While many aspects of alternative medicine are difficult for those in the health care profession to understand, most now accept the mind/body connection. They may not comprehend it (who really does?), but they accept the fact that the mind can either heal or hurt the heart.

Love, companionship, humor, forgiveness, and prayer are huge concepts. They are affordable, noninvasive, and risk free! We've known throughout history how important they are, and now science is showing it, too. Let's love ourselves—and love each other. Let's find great joy in our families and friends. Let's live in forgiveness and allow forgiveness to be the healing oil that soothes troubled relationships. Let's spend time in quiet prayer and meditation, sharing our hearts and concerns with a loving Creator.

Health truly is holistic. We cannot reduce heart health down to a few nutrients or medications that target the heart. We approach health from a whole body/mind perspective.

We'll nourish the heart with good foods, and we'll make up for years of malnutrition with a well-designed supplement program. We'll include fruits, vegetables, oils, whole grains, legumes, and other good sources of protein, and we'll drink lots of pure, fresh water.

We'll spend time walking, running, playing, skating, dancing, hiking, swimming, gardening, sweeping, or doing whatever form of exercise we enjoy. And we'll do it with a friend or family member, if possible.

We'll stop trying to be Superwoman. We'll resolve those huge stress issues and take care of ourselves so we're not depressed.

In other words, we'll love our bodies—and take care of them. Our hearts will love us for it.

Notes

Introduction

1. Peter Angerer et al., "Impact of Social Support, Cynical Hostility, and Anger Expression on Progression of Coronary Atherosclerosis," *Journal of the American College of Cardiology* 36 (6): 1781–88 (November 15, 2000).

2. Abraham Ariyo et al., "Depressive Symptoms and Risks of Coronary Heart Disease Mortality in Elderly Americans," Cardiovascular Health Study Collaborative Research Group, *Circulation* 102 (15): 1773–79.

3. Thomas Pickering, "Depression, Race, Hypertension, and the Heart," *Journal of Clinical Hypertension* 2 (6): 410–12 (2000).

4. Adam Clark et al., "Coronary Disease and Reduced Situational Humor-Response: Is Laughter Cardioprotective?" (Paper presented at the 73rd Scientific Session of the American Heart Association, New Orleans, November 15, 2000).

5. Nancy E. Adler et al., "Relationship of Subjective and Objective Social Status with Psychological Functioning: Preliminary Data in Healthy White Women," *Health Psychology* 19 (6): 586–92 (November 2000).

6. Clark, "Coronary Disease."

7. Barry Bittman, "Heart Attack Survival in Women: An Unfortunate Stereotype," *Health World Online* (www.healthy.net, 2000).

8. "Comprehensive Report on Monitoring Adherence to the NIH Policy on the Inclusion of Women and Minorities as Subjects in Clinical Research for FY98 and 99 Data" (November 2001).

9. Sarah. P. Wamala et al., "Potential Explanations for the Educational Gradient in Coronary Heart Disease: A Population-Based

Case-Control Study of Swedish Women," *American Journal of Public Health* 89 (3): 785 (March 1999).

10. P. S Mueller et al., "Religious Involvement, Spirituality, and Medicine: Implications for Clinical Practice," Mayo Clinic Proceedings 76 (12): 1225–35 (2001).

11. Guiseppe Schillachi et al., "Early Cardiac Changes After Menopause," *Hypertension* 32 (4): 764–69 (October 1998).

Chapter 1

1. Catherine Heath, "Gender Bias and Women's Health Issues," *Feminist Utopia* (www.amazoncastle.com/feminism/paper.shtml, 1999).

2. Iris F. Litt, *Taking Our Pulse: The Health of America's Women.* (Stanford: Stanford University Press, 1997).

3. Leslie Laurence and Beth Weinhouse, *Outrageous Practices: The Alarming Truth About How Medicine Mistreats Women* (New York: Fawcett Columbine, 1994).

4. Rima D. Apple, ed., *Women: Health & Medicine in America: A Historical Handbook* (New Brunswick: Rutgers University Press, 1990).

5. Gabriele Amersbach, "Through the Lens of Race: Unequal Health Care in America," *Harvard Public Health Review* (winter 2002).

6. Ibid.

7. Laurence and Weinhouse, *Outrageous Practices*.

8. Ibid.

9. Litt, *Taking Our Pulse*.

10. "Multiple Risk Factor Intervention Trial: Risk Factor Changes and Mortality Results," Multiple Risk Factor Intervention Trial Research Group, *Journal of the American Medical Association* 248 (12): 1465–77 (February 19, 1997).

11. Diedrick E. Grobbee, et al., "Coffee, Caffeine, and Cardiovascular Disease in Men," *New England Journal of Medicine* 323 (15): 1026–32 (October 11, 1990).

12. Laurence and Weinhouse, *Outrageous Practices*.

13. Catherine Fletcher, "Health and Gender Differences" (pages.prodigy.com/HYEW27A/health.htm, July 1996).

14. David B. Oppenheimer, and Marjorie M. Schultz, "Gender Bias in Medical Treatment," *The Journal of Gender-Specific Medicine* (www.mmhc.com/jgsm/articles/JGSM998/law.html, 1999).

15. Nigel J. Dudley et al., "Age- and Sex-Related Bias in the Management of Heart Disease in a District General Hospital," *Age and Ageing* 31 (1): 37–42 (January 2002).

16. Heath, "Gender Bias."

17. Mary Harper, "The History and Future of Women's Health: Challenges for the Future," seminar highlights (June 11, 1998).

Chapter 2

1. "Facts About Women and Cardiovascular Diseases," *American Heart Association* (November 23, 2001).

2. Jaume Marrugat et al., "Mortality Differences Between Men and Women Following First Myocardial Infarction (RESCATE Investigators, Recursos Empleados en el Sindrome Coronario Agudo y Tiempo de Espera), *Journal of the American Medical Association* 280 (16): 1405–09 (October 28, 1998).

3. Barry Bittman, "Heart Attack Survival in Women: An Unfortunate Stereotype," *Health World Online* (www.healthy.net, 2000).

4. Ibid.

5. Alison Pahkhivala, "Heart Disease: Not Just a Guy Thing" (WebMD.com, July 30, 2001).

6. Mary A. Caldwell and Christine Miaskowski, "The Symptom Experience of Angina in Women," *Pain Management Nursing* 1 (3): 69–78 (September 2000).

7. "Heart Attacks: Women Are Different Than Men" (www .focusoncholesterol.com).

8. "Women and Heart Disease: Here's What You Can Do Now to Avoid Heart Trouble Later," *Mayo Clinic Health Letter* (August 1993).

9. "CDC: First Atlas of Geographic and Racial and Ethnic Disparities in U.S. Women's Heart Disease Death Rates Released" (www.cdc.gov/od/oc/media/pessrel/r2k0216a.htm, 2000).

10. Charles W. Hogue et al., "Sex Differences in Neurological Outcomes and Mortality After Cardiac Surgery: A Society of Thoracic Surgery," national database report in *Circulation* 103 (17): 2133–37 (May 1, 2001).

11. "What Is a Stroke?" National Institutes of Health, National Institute of Neurological Disorders and Stroke (www.ninds.nih.gov, 2001).

12. Ibid.

13. Elizabeth Smoots, "Normal Blood Pressure for Women" (www.my.webmd.com, 2001).

14. Walter N. Kernan et al., "Phenylpropanolamine and the Risk of Hemorrhagic Stroke," *New England Journal of Medicine* 343 (25): 1886–87 (December 21, 2000).

15. Robert Berkow, ed., *The Merck Manual of Medical Information: Home Edition* (Whitehouse Station: Merck and Company, 1997).

16. "Who Is At Risk for Unhealthy Levels of Cholesterol?" (well-connected.com, 1999).

17. "Women and Heart Disease," *Harvard Health Letter* 10 (5): 1–4 (February 2000).

18. Ibid.

19. Ibid.

20. "Who Is At Risk?" (well-connected.com).

21. "Women, Heart Disease and Stroke," American Heart Association survey highlights and comparison (2000).

22. Anthony L. Komaroff, ed., *Harvard Medical School Family Health Guide* (New York: Simon & Schuster, 1999).

Chapter 3

1. Susan Lark, *Estrogen Decision Self-Help Book* (Berkeley: Celestial Arts, 1994).

2. D. C. Smith et al., "Association of Exogenous Estrogen and Endometrial Carcinoma, *New England of Journal Medicine* 294 (23): 1164–67 (December 4, 1975).

3. R. Don Gambrell, Jr., "The Prevention of Endometrial Cancer in Postmenopausal Women with Progestogens," *Maturitas* 1 (2): 107–12 (September 1978).

4. David W. Sifton, ed., *The PDR Family Guide to Women's Health and Prescription Drugs* (Montvale: Medical Economics, 1994).

5. Peggy Peck, "American Heart Association Discourages HRT to Prevent Heart Disease: New Advisory a Major Change in Medical Thought," *WebMD Medical News* (July 23, 2001).

6. Lori Mosca et al., "Hormone Replacement Therapy and Cardiovascular Disease: A Statement for Healthcare Professionals from the American Heart Association," *Circulation* 104 (4): 499–503 (July 24, 2001).

7. William L. Haskell and Kathy Berra, "Heart Estrogen-Progestin Replacement Study (HERS) Follow-up: HERS-II," *Stanford Center for Disease Prevention* (July 30, 2001).

8. David M. Herrington et al., "Effects of Estrogen Replacement on the Progression of Coronary-Artery Atherosclerosis," *New England Journal of Medicine* 343 (8): 522-29 (August 24, 2000).

9. Joel A. Simon et al., "Postmenopausal Hormone Therapy and Risk of Stroke: The Heart and Estrogen-Progestin Replacement Study (HERS)," *Circulation* 103 (5): 638–42 (February 6, 2001).

10. "Expert Commentary: Inside the Latest Estrogen Study," *Women's Health* (www.intelihealth.com, August 25, 1998).

11. K. P. Alexander et al., "Initiation of Hormone Replacement Therapy After Acute Myocardial Infarction Is Associated with More Cardiac Events During Follow-up," *Journal of the American College of Cardiology* 38 (1): 1–7 (July 2001).

12. Bruce M. Psaty et al., "Hormone Replacement Therapy, Prothrombotic Mutations, and the Risk of Incident Nonfatal Myocardial Infarction in Postmenopausal Women," *Journal of the American Medical Association* 285 (7): 906–13 (February 21, 2001).

13. "Gene Linked to Hormone Replacement's Heart Effects," *Reuters Health* (February 20, 2001).

14. Marcus Laux and Christine Conrad, *Natural Women, Natural Menopause* (New York: HarperCollins, 1998).

15. John Lee, *What Your Doctor May Not Tell You About Menopause* (New York: Time Warner Books, 1996, p. 42).

16. Sifton, *PDR Family Guide to Women's Health*.

17. CDC, "Heart Disease," National Center for Health Statistics (1999).

18. Christiane Northrup, *Women's Bodies, Women's Wisdom: Creating Physical and Emotional Health and Healing* (New York: Bantam, 1994).

19. "Premarin and Estrogens Decrease Thyroid Hormone in Women," *The New England Journal of Medicine* 344: 1743–49, 1784–85 (June 7, 2001).

20. "Hidden Heart Disease Rate Dramatically High in People with Diabetes," news release, American Diabetes Association (June 13, 1998).

21. "Headline Watch: Hormone Resistin May Link Obesity to Diabetes" (mayoclinic.com, January 24, 2001).

22. Ronadip Banerjee and Mitch Lazar, "Dimerization of Resistin and Resistin-like Molecules to be Determined by a Single Cysteine," *Journal of Biological Chemistry* 276 (28): 25970–73 (July 13, 2001).

23. Claire M. Steppen et al., "The Hormone Resistin Links Obesity to Diabetes," *Nature* 409 (6818): 307–12 (January 2001).

24. Lewis Landsberg, "Insulin-Mediated Sympathetic Stimulation: Role in the Pathogenesis of Obesity-Related Hypertension (or, How Insulin Affects Blood Pressure, and Why)," *Journal of Hypertension* 19 (3 pt 2): 523–28 (March 2001).

25. Merritt McKinney, "Obesity Hormone Gene Mutation Found in Some Obese," *Reuters Health Information* (November 1, 2001).

26. Ibid.

27. "Hormone Linked to Body Weight May Help Regulate Blood Pressure," American Heart Association (September 15, 1999).

28. H. Takizawa et al., "Gender Difference in the Relationships Among Hyperleptinemia, Hyperinsulinemia, and Hypertension," *Clinical and Experimental Hypertension* 23 (4): 357–68 (May 2001).

Chapter 4

1. C. Everett Koop, "The Signs and Symptoms of Stress" (drkoop .com, 2001).

2. Vincent Felitti et al., "Relationship of Childhood Abuse and Household Dysfunction to Many of the Leading Causes of Death in Adults," The Adverse Childhood Experiences (ACE) Study in *American Journal of Preventive Medicine* 14 (4): 245–58 (May 1998).

3. Ronald Pies, "What If Your Partner Was Abused as a Child?" *WebMDHealth* (September 4, 2000).

4. Martin H. Teicher et al., "The Neurobiological Consequences of Early Stress and Childhood Maltreatment," *Neuroscience and Biobehavioral Reviews* 27 (1–2): 33–34 (January–March, 2003).

5. Michael D. Yapko, *Hand-Me-Down Blues: How to Stop Depression from Spreading in Families* (Boston: Griffin Trade Paperback, 2000).

6. S. J. Blumenthal, ed., "The Nation's Voice on Mental Illness," (NAMI) *The Decade of the Brain* 7 (3), Arlington (Fall 1996).

7. Lauren A. Wise et al., "Adult Onset of Major Depressive Disorder in Relation to Early Life Violent Victimization: A Case-Control Study," *The Lancet* 358 (9285): 881–87 (September 15, 2001).

8. S. J. Blumenthal, ed., "The Nation's Voice."

9. John Gottman, "The Importance of Being Married," *WebMDHealth* (August 27, 2001).

10. Kristina Orth-Gomer et al., "Marital Stress Worsens Prognosis in Women with Coronary Heart Disease," in the Stockholm Female Coronary Risk Study, *Journal of the American Medical Association* 284 (23): 3008–14 (December 20, 2000).

11. M. Venters et al., "Marital Status and Cardiovascular Risk: The Minnesota Heart Survey and the Minnesota Heart Health Program," *Preventive Medicine* 15 (6): 591–605 (November 1986).

12. "Mental Health of Women," World Health Organization press release (October 10, 1996).

13. S. L. Olson and Victoria L. Banyard, "Stop The World So I Can Get Off for a While: Sources of Daily Stress in the Lives of Low-Income Single Mothers of Young Children," *Family Relations* 42: 50–56 (1993).

14. U.S. Department of Health and Human Services, "The 2002 HHS Poverty Guidelines" (www.aspe.hhs.gov/02poverty.htm, 2002).

15. Barbara L. Parry and Ruth P. Newton, "Chronobiological Basis of Female-Specific Mood Orders," *Neuropsychopharmacology* 25 (5 Suppl 1): S102–S108 (November 2001).

16. Judy Hodel, interview by author, June 16, 1996.

17. Adrian Angold and Carol Worthman, "Puberty Onset of Gender Differences in Rates of Depression: A Developmental, Epidemiological and Neuroendocrine Perspective," *Journal of Affective Disorders* 29 (2–3): 145–58 (October/November 1993).

18. Joseph Pizzorno and Michael Murray, *Encyclopedia of Natural Medicine*, Revised 2nd ed (Rocklin, CA: Prima Publishing, 1998).

19. S. J. Blumenthal, ed., "The Nation's Voice."

20. "What Are the Risk Factors for Depression?" *WebMDHealth* (2000).

21. I. Chen, "Are Your Emotions Hurting Your Health? *Health* (September 2001).

22. John C. Barefoot et al., "Depressive Symptoms and Survival of Patients with Coronary Artery Disease," *Psychosomatic Medicine* 62 (6): 790–95 (November/December 2000).

23. D. M. Baughan, "Barriers in Diagnosing Anxiety Disorders in Family Practice," *American Family Physician* 52 (2): 447–50 (August 1995).

24. Susan M. Lark, *Anxiety & Stress: Self-Help Book* (Berkeley: Celestial Arts, 1993).

25. A. Z. LaCroix, "Psychosocial Factors and Risk of Coronary Heart Disease in Women: An Epidemiologic Perspective," *Fertility and Sterility* 62 (6 Supp. 2): 133S–1339S (December 1994).

26. Chen, "Are Your Emotions Hurting Your Health?"

27. Larry Christensen, "The Role of Caffeine and Sugar in Depression," *The Nutrition Report* 9 (3): 17, 24 (March 1991), as cited in *Clinical Pearls*, 1991.

28. T. Tsutsumi et al., "Comparison of High and Moderate Intensity of Strength Training on Mood and Anxiety in Older Adults," *Perception and Motor Skills* 87 (3 Pt 1): 1003–11 (December 1998).

Chapter 5

1. Teresa T. Fung et al., "Dietary Patterns and the Risk of Coronary Heart Disease in Women," *Archives of Internal Medicine* 161 (15): 1847–62 (August 13–27, 2001).

2. R. B. Singh, "Effect of Fat-Modified and Fruit and Vegetable-Enriched Diets on Blood Lipids in the Indian Diet Heart Study, *American Journal of Cardiology* 70: 869–74 (October 1, 1992), as cited in *Clinical Pearls* (1992).

3. "Heart Healthy Diet" (webmd.com/well-connected, 1999).

4. Ibid.

5. Lars Berglund et al., "HDL-Subpopulation Patterns in Response to Reductions in Dietary Total and Saturated Fat Intakes in Healthy Subjects," *American Journal of Clinical Nutrition* 70 (6): 992–1000 (December 1999).

6. Kevin Vigilante and Mary Flynn, *Low-Fat Lies, High-Fat Frauds* (Washington, D.C.: Lifeline Press, 1999).

7. Vadim Ivanov et al., "Red Wine Antioxidants Bind to Human Lipoproteins and Protect Them from Metal Ion-Dependent and Independent Oxidation," *Journal of Agricultural Food Chemistry* 49 (9): 4442–49 (September 2001).

8. Dean M. Ornish et al., "Can Lifestyle Changes Reverse Coronary Heart Disease?" *The Lancet* 336: 129–133 (1990).

9. "Heart Healthy Diet."

10. Thomas J. Moore et al., "DASH (Dietary Approaches to Stop Hypertension) Diet Is Effective Treatment for Stage 1 Isolated Systolic Hypertension," *Hypertension* 38 (2): 155–58 (August 2001).

11. Eva Obarzanek et al., "Effects on Blood Lipids of a Blood-Pressure-Lowering Diet: The Dietary Approaches to Stop Hypertension (DASH) Trial," *American Journal of Clinical Nutrition* 74 (1): 80–9 (July 2001).

12. Iso H. et al., "Intake of Fish and Omega-3 Fatty Acids and Risk of Stroke in Women," *Journal of the American Medical Association* 285 (3): 304–09 (January 17, 2001).

13. Edward Saltzman et al., "An Oat-Containing Hypocaloric Diet Reduces Systolic Blood Pressure and Improves Lipid Profile Beyond Effects of Weight Loss in Men and Women," *Journal of Nutrition* 131 (5): 1465–70 (May 2001).

14. David L. Katz et al., "Acute Effects of Oats and Vitamin E on Endothelial Responses to Ingested Fat," *American Journal of Preventive Medicine* 20 (2): 124–29 (February 2001).

15. Anette Jarvi et al., "The Influence of Food Structure on Postprandial Metabolism in Patients with Non-Insulin-Dependent Diabetes Mellitus," *American Journal of Clinical Nutrition* 59 suppl. (1994), as cited in *Clinical Pearls* (1994).

16. Fraser W. Scott and Hubert Kolb, "Cow's Milk and Insulin-Dependent Diabetes Mellitus," *The Lancet* 348: 613 (August 31, 1996), as cited in *Clinical Pearls* (1996).

17. Frank B. Hu et al., "Dietary Fat Intake and the Risk of Coronary Heart Disease in Women," *New England Journal of Medicine* 337 (21): 1491–99 (November 1997).

18. J. David Curb et al., "Serum Lipid Effects of a High-Monounsaturated-Fat Diet Based on Macadamia Nuts," *Archives of Internal Medicine* 160 (8): 1154–58 (April 24, 2000).

19. Andrew Weil, "Good Fats, Bad Fats," *Dr. Andrew Weil's Self Healing Newsletter* (December 1998).

20. Hu, "Dietary Fat Intake."

21. Frank M. Sacks et al., "Effects on Blood Pressure of Reduced Dietary Sodium and the Dietary Approaches to Stop Hypertension (DASH) Diet, DASH-Sodium Collaborative Research Group," *New England Journal of Medicine* 344 (1): 3–10 (January 4, 2001).

22. Ann Louise Gittleman, *Get the Sugar Out* (New York: Crown Publishing Group, 1996).

23. J. Jepperson et al., "Effects of Low-Fat, High-Carbohydrate Diets on Risk Factors for Ischemic Heart Disease in Postmenopausal Women," *American Journal of Clinical Nutrition* 65: 1027–33 (1997), as cited in *Clinical Pearls* (1997).

Chapter 6

1. David Snowdon, *Aging with Grace* (New York: Bantam Books, 2001, p. 179).

2. "Niacin: Nicotinic Acid," *The Medical Letter* 33 (Issue 835): 2 (January 11, 1991), as cited in *Clinical Pearls* (1991).

3. James M. McKenney et al., "Effect of Niacin and Atorvastatin on Lipoprotein Subclasses in Patients with Atherogenic Dyslipidemia," *American Journal of Cardiology* 88 (3): 270–74 (August 1, 2001).

4. Linus Pauling and Mathias Rath, "Research on Heart Disease: An Ongoing Investigation at LPI," The Linus Pauling Institute of Science and Medicine 3 (3): 3 (Winter, 1990), as cited in *Clinical Pearls* (1990).

5. Gethin R. Ellis et al., "Acute Effects of Vitamin C on Platelet Responsiveness to Nitric Oxide Donors and Endothelial Function in Patients with Chronic Heart Failure," *Journal of Cardiovascular Pharmacology* 37 (5): 564–70 (May 2001).

6. Helga Gerster, "High-Dose Vitamin C: A Risk for Persons with High Iron Stores?" *International Journal for Vitamin and Nutrition Research* 69 (2): 67–82 (March 1999).

7. P. Knekt et al., "Antioxidant Vitamin Intake and Coronary Mortality in a Longitudinal Population Study," *American Journal of Epidemiology* 139: 1180–89 (1994).

8. K. U. Ingold et al., "Biokinetics of and Discrimination Between Dietary RRR- and SRR-Alpha-Tocopherols in the Male Rat," *Lipids* 22: 163–72 (1987).

9. Stephen T. Sinatra, "Coenzyme Q10: A Vital Therapeutic Nutrient for the Heart with Special Application in Congestive Heart Failure," *Connecticut Medicine* 61 (11): 707–11 (November 1997).

10. Morisco et al., "Noninvasive Evaluation of Cardiac Hemodynamics During Exercise in Patients with Chronic Heart Failure: Effects

of Short-term Coenzyme Q10 Treatment," *Molecular Aspects of Medicine* 15 (Fonatana D): S155–S163 (1994).

11. Detlef Mohr et al., "Dietary Supplementation with CoQ10 Results in Increased Levels of Ubiquinol-L0 Within Circulating Lipoproteins and Increased Resistance of Human Low-Density Lipoprotein to the Initiation of Lipid Peroxidation," *Biochimica et Biophysica Acta* 1126: 247–54 (1992).

12. V. Digiesi et al., "Coenzyme Q10 in Essential Hypertension," *Molecular Aspects of Medicine* 15: S257–S263 (1994).

13. Ray Sahelian, *Coenzyme Q10: Nature's Heart Energizer* (Green Bay: IMPAKT Communications, Inc., 1997).

14. H. Langsjoen et al., "Usefulness of CoQ10 in Clinical Cardiology: A Long-term Study," *Molecular Aspects of Medicine* 15: S165–175 (1994).

15. C. Leray et al., "Simultaneous Determination of Homologues of Vitamin E and Coenzyme Q10 and Products of Alpha-Tocopheral Oxidation," *Journal of Lipid Research* 39 (10): 2099–2105 (October 1998).

16. Stephen B. Kritchevsky et al., "Provitamin A Carotenoids Intake and Carotid Artery Plaques: The Atherosclerosis Risk in Communities Study," *American Journal of Clinical Nutrition* 68 (3): 726–33 (September 1998).

17. Z. R. Dixon et al., "The Effect of a Low-Carotenoid Diet on Malondialdehyde-Thiobarbituric Acid (MDA-TBA) Concentrations in Women: A Placebo-Controlled Double-Blind Study, *Journal of the American College of Nutrition* 17 (1): 54–58 (February 1998).

18. R. Sethi et al., "Beneficial Effects of Propionyl L-Carnitine on Sarcolemmal Changes in Congestive Heart Failure Due to Myocardial Infarction," *Cardiovascular Research* 42 (3): 607–15 (June 1999).

19. Michael T. Murray, *The Healing Power of Foods* (Rocklin, CA Prima Publishing, 1993).

20. M. Diaz et al., "L-Carnitine Effects on Chemical Composition of Plasma Lipoproteins of Rabbits Fed with Normal and High Cholesterol Diets," *Lipids* 35 (6): 627–32 (June 2000).

21. Gregory S. Kelly, "Insulin Resistance: Lifestyle and Nutritional Interventions," *Alternative Medicine Review* 5 (2): 109–32 (April 2000).

22. R. N. Iyer et al., "L-Carnitine Moderately Improves the Exercise Tolerance in Chronic Stable Angina," *Journal of the Association of Physicians in India* 48 (11): 1050–52 (November 2000).

23. S. Watanabe et al., "Effects of L- and DL-Carnitine on Patients with Impaired Exercise Tolerance," *Japanese Heart Journal* 36: 319–31 (1995).

24. J. W. Daily, III et al., "Choline Supplementation Alters Carnitine Homeostasis in Humans and Guinea Pigs," *Journal of Nutrition* 125: 1938–44 (1995).

25. Michael Murray, *Encyclopedia of Nutritional Supplements* (Rocklin, CA: Prima Publishing, 1996).

26. H. N. Sanders et al., "Effect of Potassium Concentration in Dialysate on Total Body Potassium," *Journal of Renal Nutrition* 8 (2): 64–68 (April 1998).

27. Robert A. Ronzio, *The Encyclopedia of Nutrition & Good Health* (New York: Facts on File, Inc., 1997).

28. Kazushiro Takei et al., "Oral Calcium Supplement Decreases Urinary Oxalate Excretion in Patients with Enteric Hyperoxaluria," *Urologia Internationalis* 61 (3): 192–95 (1998).

29. Michael Schachter, "The Importance of Magnesium to Human Nutrition," *Nutritional Medicine, HealthWorld Online* (1996).

30. David W. Sifton, ed., *The PDR Family Guide to Nutrition and Health* (Montvale: Medical Economics, 1995).

31. Pascal Laurant et al., "Dietary Magnesium Intake Can Affect Mechanical Properties of Rat Carotid Artery," *British Journal of Nutrition* 84 (5): 757–64 (November 2000).

32. Dan Tzivoni and Andre Keren, "Suppression of Ventricular Arrhythmias by Magnesium," *The American Journal of Cardiology* 65: 1397–99 (June 1, 1990), as cited in *Clinical Pearls* (1990).

33. C. B. Seelig, "Magnesium Deficiency in Two Hypertensive Patients," *Southern Medical Journal* 83 (7): 739–42 (July 1990), as cited in *Clinical Pearls* (1990).

34. S. Gottlieb et al., "Prognostic Importance of Serum Magnesium Concentration in Patients with Congestive Heart Failure," *Journal of the American College of Cardiology* 16 (4): 827–31 (October 1990), as cited in *Clinical Pearls* (1990).

35. David M. Sherer et al., "Transient Symptomatic Subendocardial Ischemia During Intravenous Magnesium Sulfate Tocolytic Therapy," *American Journal of Obstetrics and Gynecology* 166 (1)/Part I: 33–35 (January 1992), as cited in *Clinical Pearls* (1992).

36. Yves Rayssiguier et al., "Dietary Magnesium Affects Susceptibility of Lipoproteins and Tissues to Peroxidation in Rats," *Journal of the American College of Nutrition* 12 (2): 133–37 (1993), as cited in *Clinical Pearls* (1993).

37. J. Sheehan, "Importance of Magnesium Chloride Repletion After Myocardial Infarction," *The American Journal of Cardiology* 63 (14): 35G–38G (April 18, 1989).

38. Gruppo Italiano per lo Studio della Sopravvivenza nell'Infarcto Miocardico, "Dietary Supplementation with N-3 Polyunsaturated Fatty Acids and Vitamin E After Myocardial Infarction: Results of the GISSI-Prevenzione Trial," *The Lancet* 354 (9177): 447–55 (August 7, 1999).

39. Willliam S. Harris and Willliam L. Isley, "Clinical Trial Evidence for the Cardioprotective Effects of Omega-3 Fatty Acids," *Current Atherosclerosis Reports* 3 (2): 174–79 (March 2001).

Chapter 7

1. Stephen T. Sinatra, *The Coenzyme Q10 Phenomenon* (New Canaan: Keats Publishing, 1998).

2. Peter H. Langsjoen, "Introduction to Coenzyme Q10" (www.csi.unian.it/coenzymeQ/introduc.html).

3. Ibid.

4. Ibid.

5. Bruce Wilkinson, Internet interview, 2002.

6. Ibid.

7. Ray Sahelian, *Coenzyme Q10: Nature's Heart Energizer* (Green Bay: IMPAKT Communications, 1997).

8. Sinatra, *Coenzyme Q10 Phenomenon*.

9. B. Ley-Jacobs, *Coenzyme Q10: All-Around Nutrient for All-Around Health* (Temecula: BL Publications, 1999).

10. A. Sjogren et al., "Magnesium Deficiency in Coronary Artery Disease and Cardiac Arrhythmias," *Journal of Internal Medicine* 229: 213–22 (1989), as cited in *Clinical Pearls* (1989).

11. K. Overvad et al., "Coenzyme Q10 in Health and Disease," *European Journal of Clinical Nutrition* 53 (10): 764–70 (October 1999).

12. Mongthuong T. Tran et al., "Role of Coenzyme Q10 in Chronic Heart Failure, Angina, and Hypertension," *Pharmacotherapy* 21 (7): 797–806 (July 2001).

13. H. L. Sacher et al., "The Clinical and Hemodynamic Effects of Coenzyme Q10 in Congestive Cardiomyopathy," *American Journal of Therapeutics* 4 (2–3): 66–72 (Feb–Mar 1997).

14. Langsjoen, "Introduction to Coenzyme Q10" (online).

15. Ronald Arky, medical consultant, *Physicians' Desk Reference.* (Montvale: Medical Economics, 1996.)

16. Ibid.

17. R. B. Singh et al., "Randomized, Double-Blind Placebo-Controlled Trial of Coenzyme Q10 in Patients with Acute Myocardial Infarction," *Cardiovascular Drugs and Therapy* 12 (4): 347–53, (September 1998).

18. Sahelian, *Coenzyme Q10.*

19. Robert Berkow (editor-in-chief), *The Merck Manual of Medical Information* (Whitehouse Station: Merck Research Laboratories, 1997).

20. A. Gvozdjakova et al., "Coenzyme Depletion and Mitochrondrial Energy Disturbances in Rejection Development in Patients After Heart Transplantation," *Biofactors* 9 (2–4): 301–6 (1999).

21. R. B. Singh et al., "Effect of Hydrosoluble Coenzyme Q10 on Blood Pressures and Insulin Resistance in Hypertensive Patients with Coronary Artery Disease," *Journal of Human Hypertension* 13 (3): 203–8 (March 1999).

22. Rhian M. Touyz, "Magnesium Supplementation as an Adjuvant to Synthetic Calcium Channel Antagonism in the Treatment of Hypertension," *Medical Hypothesis* 36: 140–41 (1991), as cited in *Clinical Pearls* (1991).

23. Sinatra, *Coenzyme Q10 Phenomenon.*

24. Langsjoen, "Introduction to Coenzyme Q10" (online).

25. Anthony L. Komaroff, *Harvard Medical School Family Health Guide* (New York: Simon & Schuster, 1999).

26. Sinatra, *Coenzyme Q10 Phenomenon.*

27. Tadashi Kamikawa et al., "Effects of Coenzyme Q10 on Exercise Tolerance in Chronic Stable Angina Pectoris," *American Journal of Cardiology* 56 (4): 247–51 (August 1985).

28. Sahelian, *Coenzyme Q10.*

29. Shane R. Thomas et al., "Dietary Cosupplementation with Vitamin E and Coenzyme (Q10) Inhibits Atherosclerosis in Apolipoprotein E Gene Knockout Mice," *Arteriosclerosis, Thrombosis, and Vascular Biology* 21 (4): 585–93 (April 2001).

30. D. Schneider and E. F. Elstner, "Coenzyme Q10, Vitamin E, and Dihydrothioctic Acid Cooperatively Prevent Diene Conjugation in Isolated Low-Density Lipoprotein," *Antioxidant Redox Signal* 2 (2): 327–33 (Summer 2000).

31. Langsjoen, "Introduction to Coenzyme Q10" (online).

32. Sinatra, *Coenzyme Q10 Phenomenon*.

33. Langsjoen, "Introduction to Coenzyme Q10" (online).

34. Ibid.

35. Ley-Jacobs, *Coenzyme Q10*.

36. Ibid.

37. Ibid.

38. Sinatra, *Coenzyme Q10 Phenomenon*.

39. Peter H. Langsjoen et al., "Usefulness of CoQ10 in Clinical Cardiology: A Long-term Study," *Molecular Aspects of Medicine* 15: S165–S175 (1994).

40. Overvad, "Coenzyme Q10 in Health."

41. Sahelian, *Coenzyme Q10*.

42. Karl Folkers et al., "Lovastatin Decreases Coenzyme Q10 Levels in Humans," Proceedings of the National Academy of Sciences of the United States of America 87: 8931–34 (November 1990).

43. G. Ghirlanda, "Evidence of Plasma Coenzyme Q10-Lowering Effect by HMG-Coa Reductase Inhibitors: A Double-Blind, Placebo-Controlled Study," *Journal of Clinical Pharmacology* 33: 226–29 (1993).

44. Sinatra, *Coenzyme Q10 Phenomenon*.

45. B. S. Kendler, "Nutritional Strategies in Cardiovascular Disease Control: An Update on Vitamins and Conditionally Essential Nutrients," *Progress in Cardiovascular Nursing* 14 (4): 124–9 (Autumn 1999).

46. Langsjoen, "Introduction to Coenzyme Q10" (online).

Chapter 8

1. James A. Duke, *The Green Pharmacy* (Emmaus, PA: Rodale Press, 1997).

2. Donald Brown, *Herbal Prescriptions for Better Health: Your Everday Guide to Prevention, Treatment, and Care* (Rocklin, CA: Prima Publishing, 1996).

3. Jean-Yves Dionne, "Hawthorn: Effective and Gentle Heart Tonic," *Nature's Impact* 40–42 (February/March 1999).

4. J. Kuhnau, "The Flavonoids, A Class of Semi-Essential Food Components: Their Role in Human Nutrition," *World Review of Nutrition and Dietetics* 24: 117–91 (1976).

5. S. Rhanjendran et al., "Effect of Tincture of Crataegus on the LDL-Receptor Activity of Hepatic Plasma Membrane of Rats Fed An Atherogenic Diet," *Atherosclerosis* 123: 235–41 (1996).

6. Xiao-Hua Zhang et al., "Gender May Affect the Action of Garlic Oil on Plasma Cholesterol and Glucose Levels of Normal Subjects," *Journal of Nutrition* 131 (5): 1471–78 (May 2001).

7. Benjamin H. Lau, "Suppression of LDL Oxidation by Garlic," *Journal of Nutrition* 131 (3s): 985S–988S (March 2001).

8. S. Phelps and W. S. Harris, "Garlic Supplementation and Lipoprotein Oxidation Susceptibility," *Lipids* 28 (5): 475–77 (May 1993).

9. Thibaut Liebgott et al., "Complementary Cardioprotective Effects of Flavonoid Metabolites and Terpenoid Constituents of Ginkgo Biloba Extract (Egb 761) During Ischemia and Reperfusion," *Basic Research in Cardiology* 95 (5): 368–77 (October 2000).

10. J. Shen et al., "Effects of EGB 761 on Nitric Oxide and Oxygen Free Radicals, Myocardial Damage, and Arrhythmia in Ischemia-Reperfusion Injury In Vivo," *Biochimica et Biophysica Acta* 1406 (3): 228–36 (April 28, 1998).

11. H. Yokogoshi and M. Kobayashi, "Hypotensive Effect of Gamma-Glutamylmethylamide in Spontaneously Hypertensive Rats," *Life Sciences* 62 (12): 1065–68 (1998).

12. G. Walsh, "Tea and Heart Disease, *The Lancet* 349: 735 (March 8, 1997).

13. Stephen J. Duffy et al., "Short- and Long-Term Black Tea Consumption Reverses Endothelial Dysfunction in Patients with Coronary Artery Disease," *Circulation* 104 (2): 151–56 (July 2001).

14. J. B. Paquay et al., "Protection Against Nitric Oxide Toxicity by Tea," *Journal of Agricultural and Food Chemistry* 48 (11): 5768–72 (November 2000).

15. "Ask the Mayo Dietitian," *Mayo Clinic Health Oasis* (1999).

16. H. Hikino et al., "Antihepatotoxic Actions of Ginsenosides from Panax Ginseng Roots," *Planta Medica* 52: 62–64 (1985).

17. Thomas S. C. Li, "Medicinal Values of Ginseng," *The Herb, Spice, and Medicinal Plant Digest* 14 (3): 1–5 (Fall 1996).

18. C. N. Gillis, "Panax Ginseng Pharmacology: A Nitric Oxide Link?" *Biochemical Pharmacology* 54: 1–8 (1997).

19. Michael T. Murray, *The Healing Power of Herbs* (Rocklin, CA: Prima Publishing, 1995).

20. David W. Sifton, ed., *The PDR Family Guide to Women's Health and Prescription Drugs* (Montvale: Medical Economics, 1994).

21. Varro Tyler, "The Honest Herbalist: The Bright Side of Black Cohosh," *Prevention* 76–79 (April 1997).

22. David Hoffman, *The New Holistic Herbal* (Shaftsbury, Dorset, UK: Element Books, 1995).

23. Mark Messina, "Guidelines on Soy Usage," *International Journal of Integrative Medicine* 1 (5): 40–41 (September/October 1999).

24. Steven Foster, "Black Cohosh—*Cimicifuga Racemosa*," *Botanical Series*, no. 314 (Austin: American Botanical Council, 1998).

25. Robert A. Ronzio, *The Encyclopedia of Nutrition & Good Health* (New York: Facts on File, Inc., 1997).

26. Scott Washburn et al., "Effect of Soy Protein Supplementation on Serum Lipoproteins, Blood Pressure, and Menopausal Symptoms in Peri-menopausal Women" *Menopause* 6 (1): 7–13 (spring 1999).

27. H. Wiseman et al., "Isoflavone Phytoestrogens Consumed in Soy Decrease F(2)-isoprostane Concentrations and Increase Resistance of Low-density Lipoprotein to Oxidation in Humans," *American Journal of Clinical Nutrition* 72 (27): 395–400 (August 2000).

28. M. Rosenblat et al., "Macrophage Enrichment with the Isoflavan Glabridin Inhibits NADPH Oxidase-induced Cell-mediated Oxidation of Low Density Lipoprotein. A Possible Role for Protein Kinase C," *Journal of Biological Chemistry* 274 (20): 13790–9 (May 14, 1999).

29. Paula A. Belinky et al., "The Antioxidative Effects of the Isoflavan Glabridin and Endogenous Constituents of LDL During Its Oxidation," *Atherosclerosis* 137 (1): 49–61 (March 1998).

30. K. Linde and G. Ramirez et al., "St. John's Wort for Depression: An Overview and Meta-Analysis of Randomized Clinical Trials," *British Medical Journal* 313: 253–58 (1996).

31. E. U. Vorbach et al., "Efficacy and Tolerability of St. John's Wort Extract LI 160 Versus Imipramine in Patients with Severe Depressive Episodes According to ICD-10," *Pharmacopsychiatry* 30 (suppl 2): 81–85 (September, 1997).

32. G. Laakman et al., "Clinical Significance of Hyperforin for the Efficacy of Hypericum Extracts on Depressive Disorders of Different Severities," *Phytomedicine* 5 (6): 435–42 (1998).

33. W. E. Müller et al., "Hyperforin Represents the Neurotransmitter Reuptake Inhibiting Constituent of Hypericum Extract," *Pharmacopsychiatry* 31 (suppl): 16–21 (June 1998).

34. Jean-Yves Dionne and Sherry Torkos, *The Secret of St. Johns Wort Revealed: Hyperforin for Depression* (Green Bay, WI: IMPAKT Communications, 1999).

35. Ray Sahelian, *Kava: Nature's Answer to Anxiety* (Green Bay: IMPAKT Communications, 1997).

36. J. Gleitz et al., "Antithrombotic Action of the Kava Pyrone Kavain Prepared from Piper Methysticum on Human Platelets," *Planta Medica* 63: 27–30 (1997).

37. C. Backhauss and J. Krieglstein, "Extract of Kava (Piper Methysticum) and Its Methysticum Constituents Protect Brain Tissue Against Ischemic Damage in Rodents," *European Journal of Pharmacology* 215: 267–69 (1992).

38. J. D. Mathews et al., "Effects of the Heavy Usage of Kava on Physical Health: Summary of a Pilot Survey in an Aboriginal Community," *Medical Journal of Australia* 148: 548–55 (1988).

Chapter 9

1. Lawrence H. Kushi et al., "Physical Activity and Mortality in Postmenopausal Women," *Journal of the American Medical Association* 277 (16): 1287–92 (April 23–30, 1997).

2. Frank B. Hu et al., "Physical Activity and Risk of Stroke in Women," *Journal of the American Medical Association* 283 (22): 2961–67 (June 14, 2000).

3. Zhiping Huang et al., "Body Weight, Weight Change, and Risk for Hypertension in Women," *Annals of Internal Medicine* 128 (2): 81–88 (January 15, 1998).

4. Susan Lark, *Anxiety & Stress Self Help Book* (Berkeley, CA: Celestial Arts, 1996).

5. Nalin A. Singh et al., "The Efficacy of Exercise As a Long-term Antidepressant in Elderly Subjects: A Randomized, Controlled Trial,"

Journals of Gerontology: Series A Biological Sciences and Medical Sciences 56 (8): M497–M504 (August 2001).

6. E. Watanabe et al., "Comparison of Water- and Land-based Exercise in the Reduction of State Anxiety Among Older Adults," *Perceptual Motor Skills* 91 (1): 97–104 (August 2000).

7. Peg Rosen, "Why Cigarettes Are a Woman's Worst Enemy," *WebMD Medical News* (www.webmd.com, 1999).

8. "Women and Heart Disease: Here's What You Can Do Now to Avoid Heart Trouble Later," *Mayo Clinic Health Oasis*, 1999.

9. Thomas E. Eissenberg et al., "Smokers' Sex and the Effects of Tobacco Cigarettes: Subject-Related Physiological Measures," *Nicotine and Tobacco Research* 1 (4): 317–24 (December 1999).

10. "Women and Heart Disease," *Mayo Clinic Health Oasis.*

11. Paul L. Enright, "Smoking, Lung Function, and Atherosclerosis in the 5,000 Elderly Participants of the Cardiovascular Health Study, *American Journal of Geriatric Cardiology* 3 (4): 35–38 (July 1994).

12. Murray A. Mittleman et al., "Triggering Myocardial Infarction by Marijuana," *Circulation* 103 (23): 2805–9 (June 12, 2001).

13. Rudolph Weiss, *Herbal Medicine* (Beaconsfield, UK: Beaconsfield Publishers, Ltd, 1994).

14. Jerome L. Abramson et al., "Moderate Alcohol Consumption and Risk of Heart Failure Among Older Persons," *Journal of the American Medical Association* 285 (15): 2004–6 (April 2001).

15. Patrick McElduff and Annette Dobson, "How Much Alcohol and How Often? Population Based Case-Control Study of Alcohol Consumption and Risk of a Major Coronary Event," *British Medical Journal* 314 (7088): 1159–64 (April 19, 1997).

16. Colimbra DaLuz, "Alcohol and Atherosclerosis," *Anais da Academia Brasileira de Ciencas* 73 (1): 51–55 (March 2001).

17. "Food & Nutrition Questions and Answers," *Mayo Foundation for Medical Education and Research* (MFMER), 2001.

18. Arthur Klatsky et al., "Red Wine, White Wine, Liquor, Beer, and Risk for Coronary Artery Disease Hospitalization," *American Journal of Cardiology* 80 (4): 530 (February 15, 1998).

19. "Phytochemicals and Heart Disease," *Mayo Foundation for Medical Education and Research* (MFMER), 2001.

20. Annie Britton and Klim McPherson, "Mortality in England and Wales Attributable to Current Alcohol Consumption," *Journal of Epidemiology and Community Health* 55 (6): 383–88 (June 2001).

21. Anthony Komaroff, ed., *Harvard Medical School Family Health Guide* (New York: Simon & Schuster, 1999).

Chapter 10

1. Janice G. Williams et al., "Effects of an Angry Temperament on Coronary Heart Disease Risk," The Atherosclerosis Risk in Communities Study, *American Journal of Epidemiology* 154 (3): 230–35 (August 1, 2001).

2. Martin E. Seligman, *Learned Optimism* (New York: Pocket Books, 1998).

3. A. C. Toornvliet et al., "Serotoninergic Drug-Induced Weight Loss in Carbohydrate Craving Obese Patients," *International Journal of Obesity and Related Metabolic Disorders* (10): 917–20 (October 20, 1996).

4. Daniel Goleman and Joel Gurin, eds., *Mind/Body Medicine: How to Use Your Mind for Better Health* (Yonkers: Consumer Reports Books, 1993).

5. Mark W. Ketterer, "Cognitive/Behavioral Therapy of Anxiety in the Medically Ill: Cardiac Settings, Seminars in *Clinical Neuropsychiatry* 4 (2): 148–53 (April 1999).

6. Candace Pert, "The Chemical Communicators," in Bill Moyers, *Healing and the Mind* (New York: Doubleday, 1993.)

7. Norman Cousins, *Anatomy of an Illness as Perceived by the Patient* (New York: W.W. Norton & Company, 1979).

8. Nieca Goldberg, *Women Are Not Small Men: Life-Saving Strategies for Preventing and Healing Heart Disease in Women* (New York: Ballantine Books, 2002).

9. Adam Clark et al., "Inverse Association Between Sense of Humor and Coronary Heart Disease," *International Journal of Cardiology* 80 (1): 87–88 (August 2001).

10. David Jacobson, "The Laughing Cure," (/my.webmd .com/content /article/13/1668_50277, 2000).

11. Beverly H. Brummett et al., "Characteristics of Socially Isolated Patients with Coronary Artery Disease Who Are at Elevated Risk for Mortality," *Psychosomatic Medicine* 63 (2): 267–72 (March/April 2001).

12. M. Horsten et al., "Depressive Symptoms and Lack of Social Integration in Relation to Prognosis of CHD in Middle-Aged Women," The Stockholm Female Coronary Risk Study, *European Heart Journal* 21 (13): 1072–80 (July 2000).

13. Brooks B. Gump et al., "Partner Interactions Are Associated with Reduced Blood Pressure in the Natural Environment: Ambulatory Monitoring Evidence from a Healthy, Multiethnic Adult Sample," *Psychosomatic Medicine* 63 (3): 423–33 (May/June 2001).

14. Kenneth R. Pelletier and Steven E. Locke, *Mind as Healer, Mind as Slayer* (New York: Delta/Random House, 1992).

15. J. H. Medalie and U. Goldbourt, "Angina Pectoris Among 10,000 Men. II. Psychosocial and Other Factors as Evidenced by a Multivariate Analysis of a Five-Year Incidence Study," *American Journal of Medicine* 60 (6): (May 31, 1976).

16. Dean Ornish, *Love & Survival: 8 Pathways to Intimacy and Health* (New York: HarperCollins, 1999).

17. Michael E. McCullough, ed., *Forgiveness: Theory, Research, and Practice* (New York: Guilford Press, 2001).

18. Witvliet vanOyen et al., "Granting Forgiveness or Harboring Grudges: Implications for Emotion, Physiology, and Health," *Psychological Science* 12 (2): 117–23 (March 2001).

19. "How the Link Between Forgiveness and Health Changes with Age," news release, *The University of Michigan News and Information Services* (December 11, 2001).

20. Edwin L. Morris, "The Relationship of Spirituality to Coronary Heart Disease," *Alternative Therapies in Health Medicine* 7 (5): 96–98 (September/October 2001).

21. William J. Strawbridge et al., "Comparative Strength of Association Between Religious Attendance and Survival," *International Journal of Psychiatry Medicine* 30 (4): 299–308 (2000).

22. William S. Harris et al., "A Randomized, Controlled Trial of the Effects of Remote, Intercessory Prayer on Outcomes in Patients Admitted to the Coronary Care Unit," *Archives of Internal Medicine* 159 (19): 2273–78 (October 25, 1999).

23. Garret Condon, "Healing Power of Prayer Study: Saying the Rosary Aids the Heart" (www.catholic.net/hope_healing /template_channel.phtml?channel_id=22, 1991).

Index

abdominal fat: and cortisol, 2; and heart disease, 37–38
abuse, of children and women, 62–64
ACE inhibitors, 118, 138
acupuncture, 76
acute myocardial infarction (AMI), 5
adenosine triphosphate (ATP), 14, 133
adipose (fat) tissue, 55; abdominal, 2, 37–38; lower-body fat, 83; upper body fat, 83
adrenal glands, 53
adrenal hormones, 52, 101
adrenaline, 53, 72, 74, 168
aerobic exercise, 74, 162, 164, 169
African American women: higher risk of heart disease and stroke than women in other ethnic groups, 30, 39; unique medical struggles of, 16–17
aggression, 63
alcohol consumption, 40; dark side of, 177; and heart disease, 175–77; and hypoglycemic symptoms, 74; and magnesium deficiency, 122
alcoholism, 177
allergies, and depression and/or anxiety and panic disorders, 77
allopathic medicine, 159
alpha-carotene, 114, 115
alternative medicine, 190
Alzheimer's disease, 107
American Association for Therapeutic Humor, 184
American Dental Association, 39
American Heart Association (AHA): on estrogen treatment in postmenopausal women who had heart attacks, 46; first conference on women and heart disease, 16; on hormone replacement therapy (HRT), 33, 45–46; recommended diet, 86; on women and heart disease, 25
anaerobic exercise, 164, 170
anchovies, 89
anger: effect on heart, 180; and risk of a heart attack, 72
angina pectoris, 12, 138–39; and hawthorn, 147; in women, 28
angioplasty, 136
anovulatory, 50
antiarrhythmic agents, 142
anticoagulants, 112, 138, 139
antioxidants, 90, 110, 114, 125, 176
anxiety: and depression, 69; impact of exercise on, 168; and menopause, 68; potential remedies, 73–75; and stress response, 183; and symptoms of cardiovascular disease, 71

anxiety disorders, 69–71
aorta, 11
Appalachian region, 30
Apple, Rima D., 16
apple-shaped, 37
arrhythmias, 12, 74, 121
artificial sweeteners, 73–74, 99
ascorbic acid (vitamin C), 110
Asian ginseng (panax ginseng), 151
Aspartame (Nutra Sweet™), 73–74
aspirin, 42
astaxanthin, 114
atherosclerosis, 13; and CoQ10, 140; and hawthorn extract, 147; and high cholesterol, 139; and hypertension, 12; and lipid peroxidation, 87; and smoking, 173; and Syndrome X, 55
Atherosclerosis Risk in Communities Study, 180
atorvastatin, 108
atrial fibrillation, 40
axon, 123

bacterial endocarditis, 13
Baltimore Longitudinal Study, 19
Beardsley, Edward H., 16
Beck, Aaron T., 182
beef, 97
Benson, Herbert, 189
beta-blockers, 135
beta-carotene, 114
binge drinkers, 177
bioflavonoids (carotenoids), 91, 113–15
bioidentical plant hormones, 49
biosynthesis, 140
bipolar disorder, 67
bitterness (unforgiveness), 186
black cohosh (cimicifuga racemosa), 57, 152, 153
black tea, 150
blood clots, 82–83, 135; and diabetes, 32; and fish, 89; and garlic, 149
blood pressure: checking, 40; diastolic, 56, 74; effect of diabetes on, 38; and hawthorn, 147; health for women, 32; lowering, 137; medicines, 142. *See also* hypertension
blood sugar: balancing through diet, 59; effect of ginseng on, 151
blood vessel dilators, 142
blood viscosity, 138
bluefish, 89
body temperature, as barometer of metabolism, 58
brain hemorrhage, 13
brassica family, 59